Clean Your Clutter, Clear Your Life

. . . a practical manual
using Feng Shui principles

Gaylah Balter

Published by:

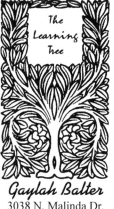

Gaylah Balter
3038 N. Malinda Dr.
Fayetteville, AR 72703
501-582-4145

Cover photo art from the "Collector's Edition" of *Birds and Blooms,* page 47. Photographer is Dick Dietrich. Cover design by Jan Cooper, Fayetteville, Arkansas.

_____

_____

Publisher's Cataloging-in-Publication

Balter, Gaylah.
   Clean your clutter, clear your life : a practical manual using feng shui principles / by Gaylah Balter.--
      1st ed.
      p.cm.
   Includes bibliographical references.
   ISBN: 0-9707861-0-7
   1. Feng shui. 2 Orderliness. 3. House cleaning--
Miscellanea.   I. Title.

BF1779.F4B35 2001   133.3'337
                          QBI01-20078

ISBN 0-9707851-0-7

DEDICATION

Thanks to my daughter, Anaya, and my son, Ariel, for their excellent editing and help in this project. They are my best critics and my best supporters. Thanks also to Ariel's fiancé, Karen, who did some really good editing, and to Alan, Anaya's partner, for support as well. I would be remiss if I did not express my gratitude to my dog, Joseph, who has taught me all about love and patience.

Thanks to my bathtub, where I get a lot of my ideas!

CONTENTS

Preface

This we know—the Earth does not belong
to man; man belongs to the Earth. ...
Man did not weave the web of life;
he is merely a strand of it. Whatever he
does to the web, he does to himself.

—Attributed to Chief Seattle, 1854*

I decided to write this book to assist my students and others who are searching for ways to get their lives to go in new directions and free themselves from procrastination, low energy levels, feelings of failure, and old emotional baggage.

For the past twenty years, I have looked for ways to bring balance, purpose, and healing to my life. In 1986, I discovered Taoism and Master Mantak Chia's work. From then on, my life took a different direction. I became a steady meditator and then a massage therapist, going on to become a teacher of The Healing Tao (Master Chia's system of self-healing). In the process, I changed my life and began to understand and use energy (**chi**) for healing mental, physical, emotional, and spiritual elements of my life and in my work with others as well.

In 1995, I began to get interested in **Feng Shui** (pronounced fung shway). This was a very natural path for me to take since, as a young girl, I bought decorating magazines with my babysitting money. My interest continued as an adult, when I studied color and interior design. As I added to my knowledge regarding the nature of energy (**chi**), all these disciplines combined to create a way for me to help others using the principles of **Feng Shui.**

My life moved in ways that taught me the value of the environment and treating the earth gently and with respect. Since **Feng Shui** teaches that all things are interconnected, it follows that what we do to the Earth we also do to ourselves. In addition, I began to understand that having so much "stuff" was one of the ways that our culture deadens our sensitivity to the Earth and the irreplaceable nature of so many of the things that we all take for granted.

I assessed all my possessions, and in the last eight years, I've either given away or sold more than half of my worldly goods. My ability to be more aware, focused, and observant began to increase as I released the clutter around me. New opportunities and ideas flowed in. I no longer feel tied to anything I own and have come to realize that all things can be replaced, if needed. I learned to trust that beautiful things are always available. This new way of looking at my "stuff" has made me feel lighter, more in control, and given me a sense of freedom that I never had.

There are many other books available at your local bookstore or library by experts in the fields of cleaning, organization, strategy planning, and simplifying life that can help you further. Look in the last chapter of this book as well as in the resource guide for some of these books.

I am grateful to all my teachers for providing me with knowledge and the ability to help others: Carol Bridges, Terah Kathryn Collins, David Daniel Kennedy, and most recently Master Thomas Lin Yun.

A special thank you goes to Harriet Hamilton and Hilde Seevers who helped me examine my writing, ideas, and purpose with humor, skill, insight, and inspiration. Their input changed the book in wonderful ways. As this happened, I was able to see new areas of creativity and also my own cluttering habits. This process created healing for me as I was writing my book. Thank you to Cindy Downs for helping me understand my computer. Without Jan Cooper, my wonderful editor, this book would not have been printed. She midwifed it as one would assist in birthing a baby. I am so grateful for her expertise and gentle nurturing.

Many of my students who also offered help and advice are Patty Heller, Judith Tavano, David Wilson, Mary Lightheart, Debi Lambeth, and Connie Monticello. Thanks to all of you and to other students who asked questions in workshops and made comments that inspired me to think about things differently and gave me ideas for this book.

Well, let's begin our journey together.

*My research has shown that Chief Seattle did not say the words attributed to him in 1854 and printed in this Preface. It is believed that Ted Perry, a screenwriter for a documentary about the environment, wrote the words in 1972 that have been attributed to Chief Seattle. It is an ecological message of universal brotherhood, rather than a haunting message about the deep gulf between the Indians and Europeans of Chief Seattle's real speech in 1854. (Taken from the Internet: www.chiefseattle.com/history/chief/seattle/speech.htm.)

How to Use the Visualization at the End of Each Chapter

At the end of each chapter, I have included a visualization related to the topics in the chapter. This is intended to help you understand and activate these ideas. Visualization has been used for millennia as another form of meditation and is known to reduce stress and anxiety and increase self-esteem. It is a process of picturing what you want in your mind and then seeing it happen.

Remember that you are in a meditative state when visualizing. It is important that you enter this state properly by taking three cleansing breaths in through your nose and out the mouth. This gets rid of old, stale, toxic material and immediately establishes a meditative state of mind. It is also recommended that you provide a quiet and uncluttered spot for yourself. If possible, turn down the ringer on your phone(s) or close the door. Always end the visualization with a positive message to yourself, then open your eyes and come back.

You might find it helpful to record each visualization on tape and then play it back to yourself as you sit with your eyes closed. Listening to the material in each visualization frees you to concentrate on the images, feelings, and ideas presented and then to use them as you wish.

Chapter 1

In the Beginning, There Was Clutter

*. . . for in the Taoist view there really is no obdurately
external world. My inside arises mutually with my outside,
and though the two may differ, they cannot be separated.*

—Alan Watts, *Tao: The Watercourse Way*

This book is designed to be a quick reference guide on
how to clean clutter, how to understand the meaning of clutter
in your life, and how to use **Feng Shui** principles to energize
the whole process. Here is an overview of what you can expect
to find in the following chapters.

STEPS FOR SUCCESSFUL CLUTTER CLEANING

- Understanding and defining all aspects of clutter.
- Awareness of different kinds of clutter and their
  effects.
- Tools to lift your personal and environmental energy
  (**chi**).
- Ways to assess your clutter.
- Ways to start your first project and stay clutter free.
- How to use **Feng Shui** to expand and energize the
  process.

Clutter creates anxiety, stress, and tension. Are you sick and tired of being sick and tired? The best way to make any dents in your mess is to become educated. By that I mean get to know everything there is to know about clutter. What is clutter, why do people create clutter, where does clutter show up, how does clutter get out of control, and who creates clutter. In "clutterspeak" that means: *I'm overwhelmed. Get me out of this!"*

Well, here goes. Nobody ever said you had to be perfect. Translated into "clutterspeak" again, that means whatever you accomplish in your goal to be more free of clutter will be fine. One step in the right direction is a step forward, and that's great. It's going to take courage, and you may take baby steps at first. Congratulations for embarking on this journey. You will discover even more skills as you progress with your work. I did say work, didn't I? Well, maybe. Let's call it aversion therapy. We all hit bottom sometimes. This is your recovery manual.

Let's see if things are as bad as you think they are. Following is a list of items that you can use to determine just how much clutter there is in your life. All of us experience one or more of these, so be easy on yourself. It is just intended to be an eye-opener.

Many of the books in the resource guide provide other lists or questionnaires like this one.

CLUTTER QUESTIONNAIRE

- Does it take you more than ten minutes to unearth an important document, a bill, a paid bill, or anything of importance? Y_ES_N__
- Are there papers on your desk that you haven't looked at in more than a week? Y_ES_N__
- Has a utility ever been turned off because you forgot to pay the bill or misplaced it or the reminder? Y__ N_o_
- Do newspapers and magazines pile up unread? Y_es_N__
- Do you frequently procrastinate so long on a work assignment that it becomes an emergency or panic situation? Y_es_N__
- Has anything been misplaced in your home for longer than two months? Y_es_N__
- Do you often misplace keys, glasses, or other important items? Y_es_N__
- Do things mass up in corners, closets or on the floor because you can't decide where to put them? Y_es_N__
- Do you want to get organized, but everything is in such a mess that you don't know where to start? Y_es_N__
- Do you save broken things for years, never repair them, and then realize that you don't need them anyway? Y_es_N__
- Do you buy things you already have? Y_es_N__
- Under your sink are there numerous "miracle" cleaners that you have never used? Y_es_N__
- Do you have spare parts to unknown things? Y_es_N__
- Do you keep putting things in places that you know aren't right, then tell yourself you are setting them there just for now? Y_es_N__
- Do you feel that your storage problems would be solved if you had more space? Y_es_N__
- Do you live in a house with more storage space than you've ever had, yet you still don't have enough? Y_es_N_o_ _don't know_
- Do you feel guilty and depressed about the state of your home or office? Y_es_N__
- Would you entertain more often if only you could get things under control? Y_es_N__

Did reading this list get you to start thinking, and did you say yes to more than ten questions? You are not alone. There is hope for you. You are now aware of many areas of clutter in your life. Together, we can set out to change the situation for the better. I have some great tools for you, so read on and don't get discouraged. Keep a sense of humor about clutter, and while you work, take care of yourself and start a journal of your clutter cleaning process. You can use the journaling pages provided at the end of each chapter. Referring to a record of what you have accomplished will be very helpful on your journey of change.

We live in a culture that constantly sends messages to buy, to acquire, to collect, to own, and to desire more of everything. We find ourselves unable to stop. We shop, then come home only to discover that we already have, stuck under a pile, the very thing we have just purchased. Or we find there isn't any more room in the shed, garage, attic, basement, or closets. In fact, we can't even go into some rooms because our passage is blocked by piles of paper, books, unopened mail, newspapers, magazines, or soiled clothing. *(Are you wondering: "How did she know I can't get around my house with my new scooter?")*

Our homes are so filled with clutter that it is difficult to clean them, and the disorder is always on our minds, making us anxious and depressed. We feel weighed down, exhausted, and helpless at the thought of doing something about the mess. Weeks follow weeks and become months. We feel worse. Our self-respect and self-esteem are constantly being eroded by our homes and workplaces — the very places that should be nurturing and supporting us.

In this book you will learn how **Feng Shui** uses clutter cleaning as a way to bring forward movement and expansion into your life. You will also learn how **Feng Shui** can transform your physical environments into supportive, harmonious, and nurturing places, and create a gathering place for the goodness of life to come forth. You will become aware of the elements in your home/workplace/life that are out of balance and are causing chaos. With this knowledge in your hands, you will be able to change your present random approach to life to one filled with conscious choices.

My goal is to help you to view clutter cleaning not as a horrific chore that you constantly put off, but as a transformational experience that will in the end release negative emotions, generate more energy, and allow you to create what you want in your life.

You will begin to understand why clutter drains your energy, prevents you from achieving your goals, blocks your vitality, affects your health, and even limits your relationships and opportunities. I will also present the idea that your physical, emotional, mental, and spiritual domains are all connected and are in turn influenced by everything around you in your immediate environment. These concepts represent the wisdom of **Feng Shui**.

I have refrained from using words that express war, fighting, or battles. Our culture seems to be focused on these words. They are used to express ideas and feelings that have nothing to do with their real meanings. For example, people say, "I just **love** him/her to death." They mean that they have so much love for the person that expressing it is difficult. Not saying what you really mean confuses your communications and you.

Words that express war, fighting, or battles pop up regularly to describe just about anything in the media, in literature, and in our figures of speech. This is a dangerous trend. I think our children are influenced by this manner of speech, and it increases the amount of violent expression in our society.

Language is used to describe feelings, thoughts, and ideas. What you say has power and can influence you and others positively or negatively. Ask yourself if any of the following words really express how you feel and the message you wish to send in the situations that you use them. Some of these words are: kill, attack, battle, deal a blow, assault, fight, war, combat, shoot down, blast away. I believe they get in the way of calming, harmonious, and positive thoughts that are necessary for the work you have set out to do, so try to eliminate them from your communications.

Let's go on with discovering more about the effects of your cluttering habits. I am hoping the following story helps to make you more aware of and sensitive to your surroundings and to the effect they have on your life. To do this, we are going to meet Rebecca, a typical career woman, retired person, or stay-at-home mom who is devoted to her work. I am sure men can relate to her story as well. Her nerves are always frazzled, and she has little time or energy to reflect on her life. Let's look at a typical day.

Awakened by her clock/radio, Rebecca goes in to take a shower and can't seem to find her shampoo because she did not return it to its usual spot yesterday. Wasting precious time and tripping over her hair dryer cord (which also hadn't been returned to its place), she proceeds to shower. She dries herself with a damp, musty towel because there are no clean ones available. Already feeling the day is starting badly and noting to herself that almost every day starts this way, she makes her way to her closet to find something to wear. The suit she wants to wear is not in its place, and its skirt has become separated from the jacket. More precious time is wasted looking for a blouse to wear as she realizes the one she likes isn't pressed. She feels guilty about the condition of her closet and distressed that so many difficulties occur even before she gets to work.

Breakfast has to be quick because there isn't enough time to fix anything nutritious. She arrives at the office barely in time for a very important appointment. Her brain isn't functioning well, due in part to the sweets she ate for breakfast, and the meeting does not go well. The rest of the day follows the same pattern. Her desk is a mess, and an important document cannot be found. Nothing solid is accomplished because she has trouble concentrating and the pile-up on her desk leads to the procrastination of important work. Relationships with her colleagues feel rushed and disjointed.

Rebecca gets home after her drive from the office and notices that an oil change is long overdue for her car. She attempts to start cooking dinner and discovers that there is really nothing in the pantry or fridge, and the piles on the counters are very irritating, leaving hardly any space to prepare a meal. She finally calls for a pizza as she has done once a week for the past month. In the evening, she decides to work on her income taxes but cannot find all the appropriate documents. She climbs into bed exhausted, nerves all a-jangle, and with that awful feeling that her day went badly and that the same thing will probably happen all over again tomorrow.

If this story applies to you completely or in a small way, take heart! There's hope around the corner. Many things are contributing to the annoying and stress-producing events that cause Rebecca so much pain and frustration. Following are some suggestions to help change the patterns that Rebecca and possibly you have allowed to take hold.

Making Some Changes

- Hanging up your towels as you use them allows them to dry for use the next day. Family members can learn to do this as well. Americans wash too many things before they are really dirty.

- Recently on the news it was reported that Americans are just too clean and that children need more exposure to dirt in order to boost their immune system's ability to respond to germs. Naturally, it is important to have good cleaning habits around the kitchen counters and in the handling of food, etc. Many people have started changing their towels only once a week or even longer and their sheets perhaps every two weeks. After all, you are clean when you dry yourself and the bed can be freshened each day in just a few minutes. (See my quick bed-making technique in Chapter 9.)

(No, that's not all. →)

- Creating lists of the foods you need for quick and appealing meals will make shopping easier.

- Creating to-do lists will help you remember the things that are important for you. You can't remember everything; it is too taxing for your brain, so to-do lists are the way to go. This will give you more control over your life and lessen the tensions.

- I also recommend keeping a separate notebook of your goals, desires, to-do lists, and anything else you want to remember.

- Putting things back in their places and providing a place for each thing will cause a whole category of irritants to disappear

As you institute some of the suggestions in this book, you will notice a decrease in the anxiety, stress, and frustration that continually plague you. Did you notice how each event added to the previous one creating a nerve-racking combination of situations for Rebecca. Changing just one pattern can change the whole day.

We will leave Rebecca and the questionnaire and go on to defining the many aspects of clutter, **Feng Shui**, and **chi**. These definitions will help you to understand the causes and meanings of clutter in your life.

Review of Topics Covered

- Clutter questionnaire.
- Rebecca's story.
- Some changes to institute.
  - Hang up towels after each use.
  - Review laundry practices.
  - Create to-do lists.
  - Make lists of foods to keep on hand for quick meals.
  - Provide a place for everything and put things in their assigned places.

Visualization for Chapter 1
A Place for Everything

Sit down in a uncluttered area of your home. Create a quiet space by closing the door or turning off the ringer on your phone(s). Take three deep breaths in through your nose and out through the mouth. This gets rid of old, stale, and toxic material and immediately establishes a meditative state of mind.

Begin to visualize or imagine in your mind Rebecca's scenario. Do you remember how frazzled she felt most of the time? We are going to change those feelings to relaxed, calm, and positive.

Visualize waking up and finding everything you need to start the day easily and quickly. Your towels are dry, your shampoo is right where you need it, your clothes are available, and oh, the day is beginning so positively. Ready for breakfast, you find foods that you like and prepare a nutritious meal. Surveying your kitchen, you notice that the counters are neat, and the pantry and fridge are well-stocked with foods that you prefer. You arrive at work well in advance of your scheduled appointment, find your papers easily from your clean desk, and proceed to please your client. The day passes pleasantly, leaving you feeling energized, hopeful, and confident.

You arrive home to find everything you need. Remembering to look at your to-do list, you see that you are to make an appointment for an oil change tomorrow. The evening goes well. All your tax documents are now in one folder waiting for you to go over them, and you get your taxes done in a few hours. You have time for a relaxing bath and notice that all your towels are neatly folded and ready for use. The patterns they create all lined up make you feel proud of your recent accomplishments.

You slip into your pre-made bed knowing that you will have a restful night's sleep. Before falling asleep, you congratulate yourself for the progress you have made in your life and in transforming a chaotic and clutter-filled home to one that supports and nurtures you. Having a place for everything and keeping everything in its place has made the difference. You can now look forward to opportunity and good luck flowing in.

Slowly open your eyes. You are energized by all the order in your life.

Journaling Ideas

- Take the questionnaire.
- Pick three things that you can work on from the questionnaire.
- Write your own Rebecca story.
- Ask yourself if there are any messages from our culture to which you are listening.
- Write down any language you use that is not expressive of your true feelings and also those words you use that express war or battle images.

_____

_____

_____

_____

_____

_____

_____

_____

_____

_____

_____

_____

_____

_____

_____

_____

_____

_____

_____

_____

_____

_____

Chapter 2

Feng Shui and Chi Defined

Rosie Clark's Story About Clutter

Rosie Clark is a very funny woman whom I have met many times at various Dowsing Conferences. She told me the following:

> *For 18 years I stored just about anything and everything in my car.*
> *Things just landed there and stayed on and on. It was a mess.*
> *And then I was caught in a terrible snow storm and was stranded*
> *in my car overnight. I used everything in the car that night.*

When you shop for antiques, you can "feel" the many years of use and maybe even the past user(s). You are responding to the **chi** or emanations of energy that have become part of these objects over the years. You walk by your things everyday, care for them, and even refer to them in your speech. Add to this family heirlooms and things that are used by others. These are some of the invisible cords of energy that extend from things in your environment to you all the time. **Feng Shui** describes these connections and offers ways to understand them so that you can improve your life.

Feng Shui

Feng Shui (pronounced fung shway) says that everything in our environment has a physical and psychological effect on us influencing what we experience. The goal of **Feng Shui** is to take this experience and achieve a sense of well-being and harmony through the art of enhancement and placement. Every aspect of your life is anchored energetically in your living space. Your home also mirrors who you are, who you wish to become, and how you feel about yourself, including various personal unrealized and hidden aspects.

There are fine cords of energy (**chi**) connecting you to everything in your home/workplace: furniture, books, dishes, collectibles, clothes, and even your piles of clutter. This attachment occurs because you made a choice when purchasing each item and invested something of yourself in the process. You already know how emotionally attached you can become to your "stuff." Your things are calling out to you for a relationship. But you can decide if you really want a relationship with everything in your home or workplace. Everything around you has an energy emanation of some sort that can be measured. Because your possessions reflect the qualities you desire to advance in your life, buying and having things that you truly love and nurture you will not create clutter and is good **Feng Shui**.

According to **Feng Shui** principles, nothing positive can take place in your personal life until you deal with the clutter. This Chinese wisdom teaches how to encourage the unobstructed movement of **chi** (lifeforce) in your environment so that it benefits the physical, emotional, mental, and spiritual aspects of your life. The entrance to your home/workplace is the gateway of **chi**, so clearing any obstructions to this flow is wise. Using the time-tested principles of color, placement, and enhancement, you can bring the qualities of balance, freedom, clarity, harmony, increased energy, health, and prosperity into your life. You can make changes in your home and workplace that reflect the changes you want to make in your life.

Feng Shui offers ways to conceptualize and formalize common sense inspired by years of observation, trial and error, and folk wisdom. When adding **Feng Shui** to the mix of modalities used, understanding is deepened and the number of possible solutions is expanded.

Feng Shui, being both art and science, brings more than 3,000 years of accumulated Chinese, Tibetan, and Indian wisdom to the learning process. America, being both practical and fun-loving, brings humor and strategies for organizing. This blend of ideas works very well together to create a body of knowledge that contains solutions for everyone's problems. There are many schools of **Feng Shui**. I follow the Black Hat School developed by Master Thomas Lin Yun of Berkeley, California.

Chi

To use **Feng Shui** effectively, knowing more about its essence will be helpful.

In the Orient, energy and vital force, or lifeforce, is called **chi**, qi, or ki. I will be using **chi** in this book. **Chi** can also be described as the living force that animates all things. It is given special names in other cultures such as: "prana," Indian; "ruach," Judaism and the Bible; "Great Spirit," Native American, and "God" in many religions.

Chi ebbs and flows like water and is viewed as the blood of the universe. Just as blood courses in the veins of all living things, **chi** flows throughout the universe bringing lifeforce wherever it goes.

Chi is everywhere, in everything (even inanimate or man-made objects), and is always changing from one form to another, says Terah Kathryn Collins in *The Western Guide to Feng Shui*. Since we live in an interconnected world, we are influenced by everything, even the unseen force of **chi** as it is expressed in our possessions and our environment. If this is so, then all the things that we select to be part of our lives ought to be carefully chosen because they have so much effect on us.

Symbols

Symbols are a very important part of **Feng Shui** and Chinese culture. Their language is formed by symbols and based on the sounds of the words and the images they create. The concept of hidden meanings plays a large part in Chinese spiritual traditions and in their art, music, architecture, and literature. Simply stated, when things are empowered with subtle meanings, our subconscious minds are stimulated. These images then have the power of suggestion. **Feng Shui** teaches that everything in our environment is imbued with the power of suggestion and that symbols work on us at subconscious levels. For instance, do you have difficulty moving around your home? This could indicate or symbolize that you may have some obstacles in certain areas of your life.

To further elaborate on this subject, I would like to share with you information from an article that appeared in 1998 in *Qi, Journal of Health and Fitness*, "Feng Shui and Symbolism," p.44-45, by Jenny Liu. She introduces the idea that images and stimuli are always activating our mental and emotional states and, therefore, influence our goals, desires, and feelings. She says that symbols impact our subconscious minds where they invoke memories from the past and stimulate our present experiences. In addition, the subconscious mind comprises about 95% of our mind, and it understands and works with symbols as its language.

Using this principle, I chose the cover on this book for its symbolic message. The spider web represents the web that each of us weaves as we accumulate clutter. Most spiders destroy or eat their webs at the end of the day, leaving no clutter. The flowers on the cover represent the future, which unfolds each day with such innocence and promise.

Intuition

The third aspect of **Feng Shui** to be discussed is intuition. Whenever you are in contact with how you feel, you are in an intuitional state. It is important to value and have faith in these states of feeling since they provide you with information that is totally true for you and only you. In making assessments of your environment and your home and/or workplace, you will need to use this skill. In the future, you can use your intuition to guide you in making purchases and decisions related to clutter cleaning. I will present ways for you to be more in touch with your feelings in Chapter 7.

While living in North Carolina several years ago, it became clear to me after meditating that I should move. I had been resisting my feelings. When I examined them more carefully, I realized that my intuition was right. Since I have always trusted that my intuition was correct, why didn't I listen this time? I put up barriers to listening because of the tremendous job I was facing if I decided to move. Fear came up as I realized how many changes would occur. I felt the fear, broke through the resistance, listened to my intuition, and moved.

> **Important: Your intuition comes to you through your feelings. Trust them!**

I hope you have a clearer picture of how much you are influenced by your surroundings and possessions. Less clutter in your life will translate into less anxiety, more awareness, and increased sensitivity to symbols and to the effects of clutter. I will be using these **Feng Shui** concepts throughout the book to explore all the aspects of clutter.

Congratulate yourself for the courage in setting out on a journey, for risking and stepping out into the unknown and unfamiliar. You have demonstrated to your subconscious mind that you are indeed serious about your goal.

Review of Topics Covered

- **Feng Shui** defined.
- **Feng Shui** defined even more:
  chi, symbols, and intuition.

Visualization For Chapter 2
Symbols

Sit down in an uncluttered area of your home. Create a quiet space by closing the door or turning off the ringer on your phone(s). Take three cleansing breaths in through your nose and out the mouth. Close your eyes and imagine you are getting out of your car; this time you didn't park in the garage. I know the garage is easier, but occasionally you have to use your front door to energize the possibility of good luck and opportunity finding you. You walk down a path towards your home. You are approaching your front door.

Stop for a moment and let all the images flooding your mind come into focus. Quiet your mind and allow yourself to view your home. What do you see? Weeds, dying plants, newspapers stored on the porch along with a flimsy beach chair and lots of leaves and grimy stuff.

Do you feel welcomed, nurtured, "en-tranced," and invited in? Are you proud of what you see? Does it pull your energy down, make you feel self-conscious and a little embarrassed? Is it how you would like it to look? What are the symbolic meanings of all the things that you see everyday?

Could weeds represent things clogging your life? A flimsy chair could mean lack of support, and papers and dirt could symbolize lack of attention to details, neglect, and procrastination. What can you do to correct the situation? You could replace the chair with two sturdy chairs and a table for two and see if support and improved relationships develop.

You could clean up the mess to discover that new ideas and opportunity occur soon.

These solutions are also a common sense approach. **Feng Shui** enhancements often take this direction. Cleaning up a mess and providing sturdy chairs will change any environment for the better. We can take this to a different level using the **Bagua**. If your front entrance is in the career area, then the weeds, grime, and neglect could symbolize a career that is stuck as well as symbolizing procrastination around making changes.

Your work took twenty minutes, far less time than you thought. You find yourself at your local garden center buying some annuals to place near your front path. They provide a welcoming addition.

Now, come in again and walk up your path to the front door. Do you feel any different? Yes, it's so clean and pleasant. It seems to say you are looking at your path in life with more hope and less anxiety. It seems to say to you and to the world that you have changed and your entrance reflects these changes. You have experienced first hand the power of symbols. You are confident, calm, and happy.

Journaling Ideas

- Look at your relationship with your things. Select three items and determine how you are influenced by them, what they symbolize, and what kind of energy they emit.
- Note three ways you can become more aware of your feelings (intuition).
- Note some ways you observe **Feng Shui** to be working in your life.

Chapter 3

Clutter Defined and Why People Hold Onto Their Clutter

Rabbi Joseph was sitting in his study when a traveler came through his village and paid a visit. He looked around the room and declared, "Rabbi why don't you have any possessions?"

The Rabbi looked up from his studies and replied, "You don't have anything with you either."

"Well, I am just passing through," said the traveler

Rabbi Joseph looked up and said, "I am, too."

—Author Unknown

People hold onto clutter for many reasons, sometimes they don't even remember why. They conveniently forget about the piles and go on to something else. It is just too hard, too exhausting, too anxiety-producing to address.

In this chapter, I have collected many of the reasons why people keep clutter. You may have more to add. I remind you at this time to write these in your journal at the end of the chapter. Please keep a sense of humor about these reasons since everyone has done at least one. Yes, me too. Laughing at ourselves when we get too serious is good. I needed some comic relief so I decided to inject humor into as many places in this book as I could. Go along with it and humor me. Ok, I'll stop for now.

Clutter Defined

- In Old English, clutter is defined as a "lump or a clot." Dictionaries define clutter as a "crowded and untidy collection of things."
- According to **Feng Shui**, clutter is stuck energy appearing in many forms. Let's examine them.
- Clutter is created when things are disorganized or mixed together, don't have a place of their own, or are not returned to their places.
- Things that are neglected such as putting off repairs, servicing of appliances, or not returning phone calls are other forms of clutter. This includes things that are not wanted, are unloved, or unused.
- Too many things in a small space create a home/workplace that can't breathe, restricting the flow of beneficial **chi**. This can show up as constipation, congestion, clogged skin, and constriction.
- Chronic procrastination, and things left unfinished, or pushed aside cause other forms of clutter.
- Clutter can form as an outward symptom of what is happening in your life at the moment.

Those piles which you avoid and make you feel uneasy are also anxiety-producing. In fact, just knowing areas of your home or office are filled with clutter causes tension and worry. Feel the discomfort. Until you dislike the mess enough, you won't seek change. So discomfort is good, very good.

There appears to be a resonance or energy transfer occurring from your clutter to you. This means that clutter creates energy blockages and tension which translates into spheres of your life as impediments to greater abundance, health problems, and reduced energy and harmony.

Feng Shui principles have already helped you understand clutter on deeper levels. Now, on to exploring why people hold onto their clutter.

Why, Why, Why, Oh Why Do People Hold Onto All That Clutter?

I have come up with some really sick and disgusting reasons. Are you ready for this? People have many reasons for keeping clutter that prevent them from reaching out and touching themselves. Oops, did I say that? You know what I mean.

Just In Case

Some keep things because they might need them someday or 'just in case.' This is part of poverty consciousness thinking. Maybe you or your parents grew up in the great depression and have retained this outlook on life. Also, remember going to Grandma's and being told, "Waste not want not," or "It's a sin to throw anything away." These messages stuck with you and now you act on them without thinking and end up with a basement full of stuff you either don't need or desire. It would be wise to reconsider these memories, thought forms, and directives from well meaning relatives. *(I am going to reconsider my relatives.)*

Money's Worth

People like to hold onto things even if they are broken or no longer useful because they have to get their money's worth. This attitude is filled with negative connotations such as; doubting one's ability to get replacements or feeling guilty due to voices from family and the past that advised never to throw or give something away until it is used up or not serviceable any longer. Could we be living with someone else's values? *(Isn't that better than living with their stuff?)*

Appearances

Some keep things for appearances, because they have been in the family for a long time, or to satisfy a gift giver. If Aunt Velma gave you the gilded mirror on your mantle and you are keeping it there just in case she comes to visit, then where do honesty and happiness fit in? Every gift comes with the unwritten code that you can do what you wish with it. If you feel uncomfortable by seeing it every day, Aunt Velma would understand any honest explanation for not displaying the mirror. Dishonesty with yourself and the giver causes anxiety and dissonance in your life as well as contributing to a drain on your energy.

Buying things for their fashion, fad, status value, or because they might come back into fashion is very common in our culture. You are giving your personal power away if you are doing this to fit in or seek approval.

Is more better? Is bigger better? Many of us believe both are better because we have issues related to security, scarcity, and self-esteem. In our culture we are often valued by how much we own or possess. People are overwhelmed by their stuff; their possessions are possessing them. How many TV's, stereos, boots, sneakers or toys do we and our families need to be happy? Do we really want a relationship with that many things? They become a distraction for discovering more about ourselves and a substitute for relationships and intimacy. *(Can I use my Victoria's Secrets catalog instead?)*

Buffers

Keeping clutter around provides a buffer to suppress feelings and issues. Holding onto things for others such as children or grandchildren is a touchy subject. What if they never desire all those things you've saved? Some items are worth saving for future generations and because they are beautiful, meaningful, or irreplaceable. After a divorce or other life changes, it is wise to separate yourself from things that continually remind you of your unhappy past. This will help you with your future and is a positive step for you to take. I have had many students breathe a sigh of relief and thank me for reminding them of these ideas. They just needed a push to either ask their children, family, or friends to pick up their stuff and to sell or give away the rest. *(Now they don't know what to do with the empty space.)*

Obsessive/Compulsive Disorders

Many people suffer from obsessive/compulsive disorders (OCD) and it is a serious issue. A lot of energy is used to avoid dealing with or suppressing the problem. Sandra Felton is the only author writing books on clutter and organizing (see the resource guide) that I know of who deals with this issue. I had a student who told the class she had ten years of mail in boxes (excluding some bills) that she was unable to discard even though she felt uncomfortable about it all. If she had not missed what was in the boxes up to now, do you think she would miss anything if she recycled the whole lot?

Reckless shopping habits, the need to buy, have, and store things that one can't use up in ten lifetimes is problematic and needs healing. People who hoard are called packrats and it is reported that millions of Americans suffer from this. *(It doesn't seem to bother the mice — packrats.)*

Attention Deficit Disorder

Attention Deficit Disorder (ADD) is a tremendous problem in our society, especially in the schools. I was talking with a friend, and we decided that each of us had a little of this. We laughed about it, yet many people report having difficulties with attention span, reversing letters, and being severely disorganized. Maybe it's in the water? No, really, get help if you suspect you might have it. I learned from Sandra Felton's books that ADD and OCD sufferers have problems with clutter because of their syndrome (see the resource guide).

Procrastination

Procrastination can also become a serious illness if allowed to run your life and careen out of control. See Chapter 5 for more information. Procrastination, or leaving things piled up, pushed aside, or unfinished can cause a reduction in self-esteem, which is also a sign of neglect for yourself.

Deciding whether we want a relationship with everything in our homes/workplaces/life will produce a life lived purposefully, intentionally, deliberately, and consciously, according to Elaine St. James in *Living the Simple Life*. Living consciously is one of the basic principles of **Feng Shui**. Not doing this tends to create clutter.

I have presented all the reasons for cluttering that I could think of, and now I have a tremendous headache. You may come up with many more, then you can have the headache. Please jot them down in the journal at the end of the chapter. I hope it hasn't become as overwhelming as your clutter is; that was not my intention. Ha, Ha. In my experience, the fear is diminished and rendered manageable when we know the causes, then we can determine how to prevent this whole bloody mess and save me all the trouble of writing a book on the subject. Read on to find out even more attributes of clutter — if that is possible.

Review of Topics Covered

- Clutter defined.
- Reasons why people keep clutter such as for appearances, for approval, just in case, and as a buffer.
- Many of the cluttering habits that plague us come from issues of security, scarcity, and poor self-esteem.
- Illnesses such as obsessive/compulsive disorder, ADD, procrastination, and hoarding (packrats) needs attention.

Visualization For Chapter 3
Learning From Rabbi Joseph

Sit down in an uncluttered area of your home. Create a quiet space by closing the door or turning off the ringer on your phone(s). Take three cleansing breaths in through your nose and out the mouth. Close your eyes and imagine you are going on a trip. You have already packed your bag and are ready to go pay Rabbi Joseph a visit.

Reflecting back on reading the "Rabbi Joseph" story, you wonder how he managed to live that way. Suddenly, an idea comes to you—it's all in the attitude he had. What are attitudes? They are long-held beliefs that we don't question. They are also habitual modes of behavior, thinking, feeling, and acting. This can even extend to ways we handle stress.

Look at the Rabbi. Is he bogged down by "stuff" or by fears, fads, or fashions? Is he concerned with the need for appearances? Does he have lack of trust in the future? Is he beset with visible procrastination? No, he is not. Why? He has nothing to pull him away from his studies. He is authentic and congruent in all of his communications.

You wonder, what does he study? He studies the nature of humanity and his relationship with God. That always keeps him focused on the present and how he can be of service and do good in the world. He also has no stress. He is free to be who he is. He is, after all, just passing through.

What can you learn from Rabbi Joseph? You ponder this question. Thinking back to your home, so filled with your "stuff," you can hardly move around. Ah, yes, you make the connection finally about how your home is influencing your feelings. Your possessions and clutter are preventing you from being all you can be. They are keeping you from enjoying the present and being authentic, while adding to your levels of procrastination. Your anxiety is also caused by your fears of how to start and what to do.

You smile to yourself and begin to look at your home and your life in a new way. You have worked on cleaning your clutter; now you realize that you have to go a little deeper. Maybe you will re-read this chapter and see if any of it applies to you. It is not easy to change. You want to, though; you want a different life. You remember to keep a sense of humor about it all.

Slowly open your eyes and go about your day or evening feeling that you are well on your way to changing your attitudes and that this will open the doorway to the life you want.

Journaling Ideas

- List three reasons why you keep clutter.
- In your mind go over your things. Are there any that you don't like but are keeping anyway? List the reasons.
- Look at your self-esteem and write down anything you can do to improve in this area.

_____

_____

_____

_____

_____

_____

_____

_____

_____

_____

_____

_____

_____

_____

_____

_____

_____

_____

_____

_____

_____

_____

_____

_____

Chapter 4

How Does Clutter Affect You?

The reason we don't move forward in our lives is because of the fears that hold us back, the things that keep us from being all that we were meant to be.

—Oprah Winfrey

Openness, generosity, and gentleness: These are the qualities that Taoists associate with the positive side of fear. If you do The Inner Smile (a Taoist meditation), you can re-program or flush out the fear and invite in the positive, more helpful and beneficial emotions of openness, generosity, and gentleness. Now for the negative side of fear. Well, you know what happens if you are terrified, frightened out of your wits, or startled. Yes, that's it. The kidneys and bladder get involved. Fear is the negative emotion associated with your survival mechanism (discussed in the paragraphs that follow). You may call the American Healing Tao Association for names of teachers of this Taoist system of meditation and healing, 302-366-1225.

How Does Clutter Affect You?

Fear is one of the most powerful emotions you can experience. The fight or flight mechanism, a primal response to fear, anxiety, attack, or stress, will run its course when you find yourself in a situation that threatens your life, home, or family.

There are also pleasant sources of fear such as childbirth, marriage, moving into a new home, or starting a new job. In most instances, the situation gets handled, and your body and brain return to a more normal functioning mode. The chemicals that were produced to help you through now stop. If stress, anxiety, fear, and tension persist, the chemicals these states of mind produce continue to cause changes in mental, physical, emotional, and spiritual domains.

As you de-clutter your space, the chemical affects of fear and stress that have caused scattered and disorganized thinking, random acts and choices, and distracted you from your goals and desires will disappear. Look in Chapter 6 for **chi** lifters which can also help this process.

You become distracted because of the ongoing anxiety and stress; you feel helpless and cave in to your first feelings to pass on doing anything. De-cluttering appears to be asking you to throw away a part of yourself. You have developed a relationship and a connection to everything you own and view these things as part of yourself, so you tend to do nothing about the situation.

You may feel disgusted and depressed with the state of your home/workplace. Decreased amounts of energy and trouble falling asleep may also be symptoms of your clutter. One of my students reported that she frequently went over her areas of clutter in her mind before she dropped off to sleep. I encouraged her to visualize cleaning the clutter in each area and seeing the job completed and feeling wonderfully light and free afterwards. Replacing the negative image of piles of clutter with the positive ones of eliminating clutter gave her a more restful night's sleep, and she started her day feeling more encouraged, energized, and ready to work.

Ways That Clutter Affects Us

Health

(The following is "stuff" that you pay top dollar to a doctor to help you figure out for yourself. Yes, that's it. You are getting a bargain by reading this material. So pat yourself on the back for being such a thrifty person and read on.)

The piles of clutter accumulating in your homes/ workplaces can weigh you down and make you feel physically heavy. Hiding behind excess weight to suppress emotions and experiences and to protect you from problems is fairly common.

Physical symptoms and illnesses such as ulcers, hives, asthma, heart palpitations, and headaches can be caused by the anxiety and stress of clutter.

Dirt, dust, mold, even bacteria and fungus become attracted to clutter leading to nasal problems, allergies, and infections.

Piles to climb over and go around can create difficult passageways causing accidents, frazzled nerves, and less space for living, as well as creating a fire hazard.

Long-standing chronic clutter can drain energy reserves and cause depression which in turn diminishes the effectiveness of the immune system.

Well-Being

(I am overwhelmed by reading the following paragraphs. Stop, I need to do some yoga, breathing, or meditation. Light some candles. See a shrink. Enough with the suggestions. Let's get on with it. Plow right in and have someone hold your hand.)

Putting off working on projects because of junk being in the way can leave you very frustrated as well as dampening motivation and increasing procrastination levels. Unfinished projects hold you in Limbo Land which further intensifies your stress levels. *(Oh, gee whiz, is that where I was?)*

Many people feel ashamed of their clutter and don't want others to know the fact that they have clutter. Shame can lead to guilt and bouts of sadness, hopelessness, and defensiveness. This defensive attitude may also lead to a tendency to create dramas, make mountains out of molehills, and getting upset at imagined slights, says Karen Kingston in *Clear Your Clutter With Feng Shui.*

Clutter keeps many people operating in the past. Hidden in all that stuff lies old emotions and issues that may have been suppressed. It is very hard to free yourself from old patterns and emotions that no longer serve, when reminders of them confront you daily. You can feel the past in those piles and messes; they act as beacons of things better left alone.

There are papers, clothes, and many types of possessions that no longer express who you are now. When all available space is filled, nothing new can come into your life. You may find yourself limited to responses that don't reflect who you really are or who you would like to become.

Unresolved issues can be buried in piles of clutter. Many people use their clutter as a way of rebelling against old parental cues and disciplines. This sabotages their growth and future development and allows unresolved childhood issues to run their lives. *(I just want to go to my bedroom and crawl under the covers.)*

Coming into a messy room or opening a disorganized closet creates confusion rather than peace and comfort. This may diminish your ability to relax and feel nourished by your home.

Lack of self-confidence, self-esteem, and self-respect tends to snowball when clutter mounts. Huge amounts of time are spent diminishing your abilities because the clutter reminds you that you can't take care of your space.

Energy Levels

(I know what's in this grouping. I already feel tired; bring me a pillow and a blanket. I want to curl up and forget about it all.)
Feeling tired, sleepy, or drowsy all the time may very well be caused by too much clutter and stuff around you. It has the effect of blocking **chi** in your home/workplace and life by limiting pathways for airflow and freely moving life force. Anxiety creates tiredness as well.

Disorganization and messiness may also clog the wheels of opportunity and prevent luck and positive energy from flowing into your life's endeavors. You may be forced into thinking in old ways and in doing things that no longer serve your interests.

Extra housework is frequently created because of pressures to prepare for the cleaning lady or just getting things in order for you to vacuum, dust, or clean your own home. Clutter does seem to attract lots of dust and dirt, increasing the amount of cleaning necessary. *(Can I send the Great Spirit the bill for my cleaning lady?)*

Thoughts

(Did I ever tell you it was going to be easy? Thank God I didn't. Because it isn't. I am going to jump into my bathtub, get covered in bubbles, light some candles, and pour myself a glass of wine. Yes, now you know all about me and that I suffered from the greatest cluttering sin of all time, denial. Ah, but you can't come after me in the bathtub. Thank the Lord. I am safe.)
All the disorder, confusion, and frustration can decrease your ability to focus and remain calm and aware, leading to your making decisions that you regret later. Clutter around you can also increase indecisiveness. The lack of organization in your life begins to limit the ability to react quickly and efficiently to problems that come up.

Fuzziness and lack of clarity in thinking tends to keep nerves jangled and raw. Clutter has blocked your ability to think clearly and increased irritation levels, leading to even more chaos in your life. *(I am leaving for an extended vacation right now.)*

If you have a mess that you are coming home to, it is virtually impossible to really relax and enjoy your vacation. *(You can't even leave me alone when I am on vacation.)*

Clutter in your life and surroundings can cause distraction from more important things. When there is disorder, important matters can be distorted; your perspective can be lost. In addition, your sense of discrimination goes away because you get so used to the clutter.

Piles of things, projects lying unfinished, and unclear thinking can make you even more disorganized.

Relationships

I have the best solution for the next item. It comes from Elaine St. James. Talk with your partner about the things that bother you about his/her habits, etc. Make a list, prioritize, and do a trade relating to the things that bother you both about each other's clutter and habits. Decide what each of you are going to do to please the other. *(Elaine could win the Nobel Peace Prize for this one.)*

Fights and disharmony in families and among couples often revolve around cleaning up and the infringement of space caused by another's things.

Limitations on entertaining, reduction in social life, and loneliness can be caused by clutter. *(I thought it was because of my computer.)*

People relate to you much the same way you feel about yourself. If you always feel uncomfortable and frustrated, then expect the world to treat you this way as well.

There is less of you available for relating, seeking or

maintaining relationships, and joyous free-flow of energy. Feelings of passion and joy are blocked by the mountains of stuff and obstructed thoughts. The real you will have trouble surfacing and authenticity in communicating will be affected. *(I am going to look in my Victoria's Secrets catalog right now.)*

Clutter can de-sensitize you. There is so much stuff between you and the world that limitations can occur in listening, seeing, hearing, and touching. Such a high level of anxiety also limits relating in a natural and easy way with the world. This can limit opportunity and luck from finding you. *(Are you sure its not that my door sticks?)*

You will be able to take control and transform your space(s) by taking small steps, setting goals, assessing your stuff, and organizing and cleaning areas of messiness that you have been unable to address. Maybe you mean undress? Clutter really sucks. Reduced fear and stress levels will eliminate the chemicals triggered by these states of mind. Acting more proactively and more positively will become the norm as you realize that you finally have more control over your life.

It is nearly impossible to do something about your clutter until you know all the aspects of it *(yes, even the yucky stuff)* and how it impacts you. Getting to the hard core *(I am reaching for that Victoria's Secret catalog again)* of causes and effects is an important step in becoming free of all the entangled webs that clutter weaves. *(I really need a break now. Can I cry or call a friend for help?)*

Review Of Topics Covered

- Understanding fear.
- What are the effects of clutter?
- Understanding my attempts at humor.

Visualization for Chapter 4
Changing the Negative Effects of Clutter

Sit down in an uncluttered area of your home. Create a quiet space by closing the door or turning off the ringer on your phone(s). Take three cleansing breaths in through your nose and out the mouth. Close your eyes and imagine you are a member of the audience watching the *Oprah Winfrey Show*. You think to yourself how much you admire her for all she has done for women. Her program today is on eliminating fear.

The speaker has asked the audience members to look deeply into their lives for ways that fear turns up or ways that it has a hold on them. Instantly, you think about all the clutter in your home. You realize that you have been afraid of the changes that cleaning your clutter will usher into your life. You will have to make decisions regarding throwing away, giving away, selling your stuff. Those things that you are attached to, some will have to go. You also know that you will be looking at your thoughts, emotions, and motivations. Your suppressed fears are surfacing, and you know that something has to give because you have been in the grip of fear too long.

It is clear to you now that you have been ashamed, tired, confused, frustrated, anxious, helpless, and somewhat defensive about the condition of your home. Your life has been on hold, held hostage by your clutter. You can feel the invisible filaments of energy that connect you to every bit of it.

Imagine going home to plan your first project. It will be a small one, and you have scheduled two hours for it. You will start on your clothes closet.

You develop a plan after looking at everything in there and get a box to keep nearby, as well as a pad of paper and a pen to write anything down that is important.

Separating out empty hangars, clothes that don't fit anymore, those that need repair or ironing, and those that just don't feel right for your present life circumstances is your first task. Stopping after two hours and feeling as if it went quickly and easily once you got started, you ask yourself why you procrastinated so long. Now that you have more skills, it is easier for you to tackle tough projects, and they never take as long as you thought they would.

You are really proud of yourself as you survey the results of your work. It is so easy to find what you want, and the new order in your closet has given you a sense of more order in your life, as well as banishing any fears that may linger.

Feeling light and joyful, slowly open your eyes and go about your day or evening feeling that you are free of the fear that has been around you.

Journaling Ideas

- List some fears you have about clutter cleaning.
- List some fears you have in general.
- Look at ways that clutter affects your health, emotional well-being, energy levels, thoughts, and relationships.
- Write down some humorous thoughts you have.

Chapter 5

The Three P'S:
Personalities, Procrastinators, And Packrats

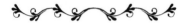

*A genuine confrontation with the truth . . . demands authenticity
and personal integrity. When one feels one way and acts in
another, one creates conflict rather then coherence and
experiences stress and disharmony or dis-ease.*

—Frances Vaughn, *The Inward Arc*

It is so important to take responsibility for your clutter.
You may feel a lot of resistance because you are asking
yourself to get rid of stuff that you have developed an energy
attachment to, a relationship with. Even though your life has
become terribly messy from all that stuff, it still is a part of
you and hard to chuck out. It appears that the more you ignore
your clutter, the more it grows, seemingly on its own.

You can do it. Keep your sense of humor, pamper
yourself, keep a lighthearted feeling going, and you will
prevail. Laughter is healing and can reduce stress as well. In
the following chapters, I will provide ways to help with this
and also some ways to drive you completely insane.

For now, let's discuss some groups of people who have
problems with clutter.

Personalities

Stephanie Winston in *Getting Organized* describes many types of personalities that mask disorder in their lives:

The busy, busy type of person lives in a flurry of activity and has little time to address their clutter.

The free spirit type of person maintains a distance from their clutter by flowing with the moment and avoiding what is around them.

The compliance/defiance type of person sets unrealistic goals, fails to accomplish them, then throws up his/her hands saying, "See I can't do it."

The guilty/defiant type of person pursues a course of action that has no effect on the people they are trying to hurt with their accumulation of stuff. They then feel guilty, and the whole process starts again.

The time warp type of person responds to forces that were in operation years ago as well as to messages from parents and family. This way of acting prevents opportunity and new ideas from entering their lives, and they become stuck. *(They are really practicing for a part in Star Trek.)*

These personality types have ways that help them avoid clutter cleaning. They put off, abdicate, or decline responsibility. They tell themselves they will do it later, then allow nature to take its course, progressing so far that their heirs have to take care of the clutter. *(Well, why not? They have more time.)*

Procrastinators

Clutter is visible procrastination, constantly reminding us of our problem. Because it is so very visible, tangible, and available it provides the very avenue for us to look at it and the people who do it — the procrastinators.

Being a procrastinator is painful. They are frequently in a panic either at work or at home (dealing with deadlines), they are not able to live in the present, and they don't have the life that they want.

"There are payoffs for procrastinating," says William Knaus, Ed.D. in *Do it Now! Break The Procrastination Habit*. Most immediately, they can go on to something else that is less stressful or distasteful. There are people who claim they do their best work under pressure. And there's the high they get from finishing in the nick of time, which can become addictive.

Procrastinators seem to be perfectionists as well (*Family Circle* 11/1/00). They feel if they can't do a job right, they won't do it at all, so they put off doing it for that perfect moment, which of course never comes. The piles of clutter mount and they do nothing. At the same time, they are afraid to be excellent because then they will have to do it all over again. This pattern of avoidance begins to limit their objectivity and awareness, and they begin to rationalize their problems.

Inwardly, they feel inadequate, so they build fortresses around themselves, such as piles of clutter. This also keeps them from being intimate. They postpone jobs and sabotage themselves because of fear of failure as well as success. It is a complex web that begins with the family of origin and is perpetuated and strengthened by our culture which sends out messages to be perfect, imposes impossibly high standards, and teaches success at any cost.

Procrastinators have poor self-esteem. As they push away, push aside, and neglect their piles and messes, their self-esteem suffers, revealing the level of neglect they have for themselves. This chain of events creates a lot of stuck energy and inertia, which is one more thing they have to work on.

Actually, most jobs end up taking about one-fourth of the time you thought, and once you get started, it becomes easier to finish. Doing the job tends to build confidence and self-esteem which in turn makes it easier to chip away at your procrastination habits.

A client of mine asked for help regarding cleaning her car. She has a very hectic life, juggling school, work, marriage, and the buying of a new home. Her car was very irritating to her and she felt that if she could just clean it out her day would start out better and also provide fewer stressors. She reported that she seemed to procrastinate and put off cleaning because it seemed like such an overwhelming job.

I suggested that she clean the car in ten minute segments as a break between other things that she had to do in her busy life. That way she could break up what seemed to be a horrendous single task into smaller, more manageable tasks, as well as providing a break from other jobs that needed her attention. She loved the idea and reported great success in the project and a boost in how she felt about herself.

Setting measurable goals, enlisting a buddy to ask you frequently how you are doing, and writing down which tasks make you procrastinate will help considerably.

Finally, list the advantages and disadvantages of putting off certain jobs or projects.

NINE STEPS TO ELIMINATE PROCRASTINATION

- Plot the entire project step-by-step and outline these on paper.
- Set measurable goals that are easily attainable.
- Make sure you have all the supplies needed to complete the project.
- Visualize every step needed to complete the project.
- Visualize completing the project.
- Do the first step immediately.
- Work for ten minutes. Now you realize it's not as bad as you thought.
- Commit to doing the project publicly. Friends will support you.
- Reward yourself liberally and find other ways to boost self-esteem.

Packrats

The packrat syndrome of hoarding has certain hallmarks. Scarcity, fear, and anxiety over not having enough are joined with never being satisfied, and always feeling lack and want as a state of mind and spirit. Those who always need to shop, buy, and spend money are also exhibiting the packrat phenomena. Packraters have problems with self-esteem and don't see abundance all around them; they see only lack. I encourage reading books on boosting self-esteem or getting professional help. This is one way to begin to understand that there is unlimited abundance and opportunity in the world for everyone.

Storing unread magazines and newspapers, little gadgets never used, endless subscriptions to catalogs, journals, and publications that go to the recycling heap before you look at them or end up in piles in your living room — all these form a barrier, a wall between you and the real world of intimacy, relationships, and communication. They keep you feeling stuffed and inundated with decisions that become increasingly harder to make.

Work with your anxiety and stress levels. High levels of anxiety can lead to panic attacks which lead to bouts of shopping to alleviate the stress and tension.

There is another aspect to this problem. I have had students who admit to having huge collections of sweaters, shoes, handbags, etc., and they say they are not upset (or won't admit to being concerned) and don't want to change. This is a whole category of problems that I just don't know how to address. I can only help someone if they feel they need it.

NINE STEPS TO ELIMINATE PACKRAT BEHAVIORS

- Find ways to ease your anxiety and state of panic. Try any of the **chi** lifters, meditation, or seek professional help.
- Resolve not to go shopping for entertainment or because you have time on your hands. Watch out for TV buying.
- Limit yourself to literature that you will read.
- Go over the literature you have now, cut out articles to save, and recycle the rest.
- Notify catalog companies to stop sending you their catalogs.
- Break up your clutter cleaning into small segments and schedule them at times when you know you can accomplish the job.
- Examine your reasons for shopping and the need for so much stuff.
- Work on ways to improve your self-esteem.
- Practice relaxation techniques every day.

The steps to eliminate chronic procrastination and packrating can be used by people in general since they offer good tips to help self-esteem, boost morale, and eliminate cluttering habits.

The following suggestions for packrats come from *I've Got to Get Rid of This Stuff* by Sandra Felton (see resource guide).

- Magnify or exaggerate your fears. They will then seem funny, and you can work with them.
- Write down your three worst problems, and then record how you would like your environment to look.
- Learn to feel where in your body the discomfort is lodged. Feeling uncomfortable is desirable and is part of the process.
- Let God have control over the future. Stop trying to control the future by keeping things.
- Come out of denial.
- Make friends with your problem to loosen its grip over you.

Review of Topics Covered

- The personality types that tend to clutter and their reasons for it.
- The complex patterns of procrastination and procrastinators.
- The complex nature of hoarding.

Visualization for Chapter 5
Changing the Energy

Sit down in an uncluttered area of your home. Create a quiet space by closing the door or turning off the ringer on your phone(s). Take three cleansing breaths in through your nose and out the mouth.

Close your eyes and imagine yourself at a very luxurious spa. You will be pampered and fussed over and provided with everything that could possibly motivate you to begin to take better care of yourself. You will take classes in exercise and taking care of your skin, hair, and nails. Experts are there to teach you how to make the best of your attributes. The food is wonderful and classes and recipes will be provided so that you can continue to eat healthfully and correctly when you return home.

Surrounded by pleasant sounds, sights, smells, and feelings, you now see how important these things are to your environment. They elevate how you feel about yourself and the world. You notice that you feel positive, energized, and happy in such surroundings, making it easier to concentrate, focus, and set goals. And you notice your anxiety level has decreased as well.

You make a promise to yourself that when you return home you will begin to institute many changes in your environment and begin to use everything you have learned at the spa in your own home and in your life. You smile to yourself because you are aware of all the good ideas presented in the chapter on lifting environmental and personal **chi**. Becoming aware of the suggestions presented in this chapter on eliminating procrastination and hoarding from your life has given you the tools you need to change your life for the better.

Three things you will do immediately are: decide on three things to clear from your home, sign up for a class in stress reduction and relaxation techniques, and let God take care of the future for you.

You are ready to utilize the suggestions because you have become aware of how they can change your mood, attitudes, and energy for doing a job that could be distasteful and anxiety-producing. You have seen at the spa how invigorating a simple aroma can be, how energizing certain music can be, how taking care of yourself, and pampering yourself can give you positive motivation.

Open your eyes and know that you can achieve all that you want to in your life.

Journaling Ideas

- List some things you exhibit of the Three P's behaviors.
- Write down three things you can do to stop these behaviors.
- Create a step-by-step approach to eliminate them.

Chapter 6

Environmental and Personal Chi

See the world as yourself
Have faith in the way things are.
Love the world as yourself;
then you can care for all things.

—Tao Te Ching

The truth is simple. You have clutter in your life because you have not been honoring your truth. It is there somewhere under the piles. You have been caught up in less important stuff that doesn't matter. You have evaded your truth. It is so difficult to do something about the clutter. Break loose from the trance and come with me to explore more meanings of clutter and get closer to your truth in the process.

Stagnating Energy

To "stagnate" is defined as "to become dull, foul, to pollute and remain motionless." Blocked energy creates clutter, and clutter then creates more slow-moving, stuck, and stagnant energy. These conditions are represented not only in piles and messes around your home/workplace, but in your thoughts, feelings, and actions. Scattered thinking, disorganization, and anxiety are their hallmarks. Let's get back to the original thing: blocked energy. Where did it come from? What started it all?

When the motifs of your life consist of random choices or a lack of conscious living, then your thoughts, decisions, and actions create barriers to the free flow of energy. As the amount of beneficial **chi** decreases in your environment, the amount of stagnant energy increases. Before long, you come to the painful realization that clutter has taken over your life, making your surroundings and thought processes cluttered. These are some of the reasons you don't heed inner guidance, don't look at painful issues, and neglect the things that matter to you. You notice you have less available energy in the evenings.

All the stuff you have thrown into piles, on tables and counters, behind doors, on your desk, on the bottom of closets and cabinets, and on top of cupboards and dressers begins to attract other bits and pieces of clutter, and the pile grows as if by magic. Then the area feels sticky, thick, heavy, sluggish, and lifeless. You skirt around the piles because they make you feel anxious and irritable. It is at this moment that you can look to the **chi** lifters in this chapter for help when you start your clutter cleaning projects.

The following environmental **chi** lifters are designed to clear the air in a room or area and create a space that fosters clear thinking, good decision-making, and keeps your resolve for work going full steam. Choose the ones that are best for you as you go through your clutter.

Environmental Chi Lifters

  ᛒ Open windows and doors to let in invigorating and cleansing fresh air.

  ᛒ Light some incense, any kind. This cleanses the air and provides a pleasant scent.

  ᛒ Light candles. Some also have pleasant aromas.

  ᛒ Bring in aromatherapy, either with a spray bottle or a bowl filled with water and several drops of essential oil set over a candle. You can use lavender for relaxation; citrus, tea tree, or frankincense for purification; and peppermint or orange for stimulation.

  ᛒ Smudge yourself and the room with a sweet grass, sage, and cedar stick. This can be purchased at your local Health Food or Herbal Store or at New Age shops. You light the tip with a match and, as the smoke rises, wave it over yourself front and back (a friend is helpful here for the back). Also wave it all over the room or zone you are working on. It is a wonderful American Indian ritual that cleanses the air and your aura helping you to feel refreshed and renewed.

  ᛒ Play music that is exhilarating, uplifting, and/or rhythmic. This will help you to keep feeling light, energetic, and positive and will bring a vibration to the area that fosters good work and helps to clear away any negative or heavy energy that surfaces from the clutter.

&ↄ Go around the room and clap, drum, or use rattles to clear and disperse the stagnant energies, old feelings, memories, or past events that come up as you clean.

&ↄ Bring a water feature or desktop fountain into the area to add a relaxing sound that will help you focus, remain calm, strengthen concentration, and humidify the air.

&ↄ Hang a windchime in the area. Used in **Feng Shui**, this acts as a symbolic element that clears the area, brings in positive **chi**, and keeps you focused. Ring it to send a message out to the world and to yourself that you are cleaning your clutter and are loving it. Ringing bells can also accomplish this.

&ↄ Hang up a faceted crystal anywhere in the room. They are used to lift and disperse stagnant **chi**.

&ↄ Wash the windows, desktop, or floors and dust, vacuum, or sweep the area you are planning to work on. This helps to clear the dirt and grime, elevates the **chi**, and in general gives you a way to start your project with tools that you already know about.

All of these suggestions are designed to help your work go more smoothly. Some of them might seem a little strange. I have found that even the most conservative professionals suggest some of them because they appear to work. Some are time-tested from other cultures and other times. Please, choose those that work best for you. Do keep an open mind about them. Remember, it was just ten years ago that aromatherapy was a strange new word, and now it's everywhere and in everything. Take the plunge and try something new.

Personal Chi Lifters

When starting on your various clutter-cleaning projects, it is important to keep your level of personal energy high, as well as maintaining a positive frame of mind. The following **chi** lifters will help you when your energy flags or you are overwhelmed with your work.

Emotions tend to surface and chaos, once a part of your clutter, will now possibly be around as chaotic feelings. Also, resistance occurs because you are chucking possessions that are viewed as part of yourself. Keep your sense of humor going. Remember, you are not alone. There are millions out there just like you.

You can do the following on a regular basis as you clean and reorganize. Some might even become part of your daily routine.

ɞ Take a quick walk. Hiking is okay, too, but of course, a little more time consuming. Getting away from the house and the neighborhood will infuse you with new energy and enthusiasm for your work. *(I may not come back.)*

ɞ Meditate or give yourself some quiet time for re-grouping. Deep breathing is part of some meditation methods.

ɞ Yoga, Tai-Chi, or Chi Kung exercises are also very helpful for relaxation, stretching, and general well-being. These classes are often offered at local hospitals, Y's, community centers, health food stores, etc. All these techniques alleviate stress that can build up as you clean.

ɞ Aerobic exercises such as swimming, treadmilling, or bicycling are good, too. *(Have you seen the clutter all that gear creates?)*

Ω Take a hot bath with bubbles, aromatherapy, and candles.

Ω Listen to your favorite music or Mozart. Mozart aids concentration and relaxes.

Ω Call a friend to help you over the rough spots. It is a good idea to establish a support system with a buddy or a friend who has agreed to talk you through difficult situations that may arise.

Ω Do some gardening. The earth is very grounding and healing and will help to infuse you with new energy for your work.

Ω Go outside and walk around in your bare feet. Take your boxes outside to sort things in the open air. This will help to give you a new perspective on things.

Ω Treat yourself to a dinner with wine at home or at a restaurant.

Ω Remember to stop and congratulate yourself for all the wonderful work you are doing. Note your feelings in the journal at the end of this chapter.

Ω Clean your house — or just one drawer. It makes you feel so good when things are in order. When you realize how little time it takes, you will be encouraged to go on and do the bigger projects.

Ω Take a break and give yourself a whole day to do nothing but errands or stay at home and dream and fantasize about how you want things to look when you are done.

൭ Watch *Home & Garden* channel on TV. Their programming is so positive, and you can also get ideas for how you would like your home to look. They do shows on closets and organizing in general.

൭ Take five to ten minutes to read an article(s) that you have been saving.

൭ Rent or go to see a good movie.

൭ Put music on that you can dance to.

൭ Buy fresh flowers for yourself and put them in the area that you are working on. They bring the same wonderful energy into a room that is contained in a garden. Flowers have energizing and healing energy.

൭ Work on a creative project that you started. Creativity is good therapy.

If you are stressed, be assured that cleaning is known to be one of the best therapies. If you feel overwhelmed, understand that anytime is the best time and small steps are good. If you feel you are too busy to tackle a project, remember that you at some point made the time to buy or order all that stuff. It is time to take responsibility for your actions. As your projects get under way, you will begin to feel renewed and your energy levels will increase.

Shoulding

I would like to offer you another way to lift your energy. Many people say, *"Oh, I should have done that."* This is called **shoulding on yourself**, and we all do it. **Shoulding** is one of the ways that you store guilt and absolve yourself of responsibility. It can sabotage all the good work that you are doing for yourself by encouraging you to revert back to old patterns and habits. Using this speech pattern feels like someone is making you do something. Experiment with eliminating **should**, **have to**, and **must** from your choice of words, and substitute *choose*, *wish*, or *desire*. Also, using the word **want** excessively implies a degree of lack. Choosing more positive words will elevate your level of communication and nurture you as well. Words have power to change your thoughts, bring in negative feelings, and drain your energy — and they have the power to do the opposite, too.

Saying No

Another great way to lift your **chi** is to speak from your heart instead of your mind. The mind will find unlimited reasons for you to say **yes** when you feel **no**. This pattern questions your integrity and increases the clutter in your life.

Contact someone you said **yes** to but didn't really want to or had second thoughts about, and cancel or say **no**. You have the right to change your mind. The new you is more authentic and honest. This is just a practice session. When you keep your integrity intact, are honest with yourself and others in all relationships, your clutter filled life will transform. You will have more energy because of fewer entangled webs of communication.

I have offered the **chi** lifters as ways for you to gain positive and relaxing time and space so work can be accomplished and to reduce the stress that can appear as you sift through your clutter. They can relieve stress and anxiety at any time, so use them regularly. These are things that **Feng Shui** encourages you to incorporate into your life to unblock the stagnating **chi**, get you moving, and bring positive thoughts and practices into existence. The next step is looking at your clutter honestly and consciously so that you can start to make decisions about it.

Review of Topics Covered

- Defined **stagnating energy**.
- Environmental **chi** lifters, such as aromatherapy, music, windchimes, water features, and washing the floor, desk, or windows.
- Personal **chi** lifters, such as exercise, music, gardening, calling a friend, treats.
- **Shoulding** and saying **no**.

Visualization for Chapter 6
The Swamp

Sit down in an uncluttered area of your home. Create a quiet space by closing the door and turning off the ringer on your phone(s). Take three cleansing breaths in through your nose and out the mouth. Close your eyes and imagine you are Jane or Tarzan in a Tarzan movie. You have lost your way in the jungle and can't seem to find your way home.

You are walking along and find yourself distracted from your situation. You smell something unusual and look ahead to an area that looks like an old pond. As you come closer, the smell gets unbearable. You see that it is a swamp and have been warned about these places, so you know what to do. You skirt the area and keep on hard ground. You think to yourself, what is a swamp and why are they so dangerous?

In the dictionary, "swamp" is defined as "an area that can suck you in and is lifeless, sluggish, heavy, slimy, decaying, and foul." You sense exactly what has been going on and why you feel so uncomfortable: Your home is blocking your energy (**chi**) and is acting like a swamp.

Clutter represents stagnating energy. What is that? It is like the swamp that you visited, only right in your home. The pollution makes you feel tired and heavy.

Now you can do something about it. In your mind, you are already making plans about some de-cluttering projects. You have decided to start with something small. You plan your project on paper and break it down into segments of twenty minutes. It is the piles of newspapers and magazines that go unread and collect dust. They must go. Beginning with the magazines, you take one and go through it. It is two years old. Zipping along, you cut out one article and put it in the file you have made labeled **To Read**. It is going very well. In twenty minutes you have only clipped six articles, and the pile is gone. You have selected the articles very carefully, noting that your interests and tastes have changed in two years. You are amazed that such a towering obstacle you procrastinated about for so long went so quickly and smoothly. This experience has taught you that you can do it again for anything in your home/workplace

You picture your home and all the areas that are cluttered and need your attention. You feel happier and lighter knowing that you can do something about your clutter. As Jane or Tarzan, you find your way home and relate your adventure.

Feeling that you will do something about your situation, you smile to yourself and open your eyes and go about your day or evening feeling that you have accomplished a great deal.

Journaling Ideas

- List ways you can make your clutter cleaning easier.
- Try one and record how it makes you feel. Record how it changed your work process and the results.
- Record ways that you **should** on yourself and ways that you can stop.
- Record ways that you can say **no** and feel comfortable.
- Write down some ways that stagnant or blocked energy has showed up in your life.

Chapter 7

The Importance of Assessing Clutter

*Getting rid of clutter is not about letting go
of things that are meaningful to you, it's about letting
go of the things that no longer contribute to your life
so that you have the time and the energy and the
space for the things that do.*

Elaine St. James, *Living the Simple Life*

Your things can influence how you feel. Do you want this connection to be positive or negative? Would you like these connections to support and nurture you? Do you desire to gain control over your life and the overall quality of your energy resources? In order to achieve these things, assessing everything becomes important.

Assessing your clutter is also important because absolute honesty and conscious awareness of all your possessions is the only way to take control, set realistic goals, and plan your objectives. Doing just your closets or your pantry is good, but that alone will not set new patterns or relieve you of the overall problem. New bouts with clutter can occur if lifestyle, patterns of thinking, and disorganization are not addressed.

I suggest that you take a walk around your home/ workplace. This will offer you an entirely new perspective towards everything that surrounds you. Walk from room to room and look at everything you own. Save the attic, basement, garage, shed, or storage unit for a later date when you are ready and have finished the work on your home/workplace.

When you decide to take this walk, you are telling your subconscious mind that you mean business. This act alone will produce changes in your life. You are at last taking action, becoming proactive, taking control. Hurray for you!

Ready? Here we go. Ask yourself the following questions as you walk from room to room looking at everything. Take your journal or a pad of paper with you to record your findings.

THINGS TO OBSERVE

- Why am I keeping it?
- What function does it have?
- Do I use it?
- Do I need it?
- Do I have others like it stored away?
- Do I absolutely love it?
- Does it bring me pleasure and joy?
- Does it inspire and nurture me?
- Is it broken, damaged, or inoperable?
- Does it bring up past memories, emotions, or negative feelings?
- What image of me does it send to the world and to me?
- Will it bring pleasure to my heirs?
- If I lost it in a tragedy, would I replace it?
- Is it outdated?
- Would I move with it five times to other places?
- Am I tired of dusting it?
- Would I place it in a special place in the **Bagua** to multiply one hundred times?

These questions ask how you feel and are designed to get you to be more in touch with your feelings and, therefore, your intuition. It is important to also prioritize the rooms you go into. Assign #1 to the most frustrating room, then assign the remaining rooms their numbers according to irritation level. Then rank the problems within each room on a list. This will help you to decide where to start. Some areas or piles will call out as being urgent or emergency situations. These get the first numbers, and the others can get the other numbers (#1 being the most urgent, and #10 being the least). Be sure to also break up the jobs into manageable units that can be accomplished in the amounts of time that you are going to set aside to do your work.

Look at all your videos, records, CDs, computer discs, collections of whatever, and books. Examine the way you store magazines, newspapers, and recyclables. Note the condition of your closets, medicine cabinets, cupboards, linens, yes, even your refrigerator (especially the doors), and under the sinks and behind doors. Peer into your filing cabinet(s) and determine if you need a new system, new files, labels, etc.

You have now been all over your house and thoughtfully looked at everything. Did it take nearly as long as you thought it would? Isn't awareness and clarity wonderful? Anxiety lessens and commitment increases. The action phase of your process has begun.

Making Changes

* Start with the most urgent area of clutter. Maybe it is the pile of papers on or near your desk, or your linen closet, or medicine cabinet, or the junk drawer in the kitchen.

- On a piece of paper begin to break the project down into manageable sections, so that you can accomplish what you want to do in the amount of time that you set aside each day or each week for your work. Of course, each project is different and will require different amounts of time.

- Write down your short-term and long-term goals in your journal, on a pad, or on the papers that you have used for your assessment walk. Writing down goals helps to increase commitment to them. Keep this part very simple. Create achievable and approachable goals.

Stop for a moment, take a deep breath, pat yourself on the back, and give yourself a big hug for all the wonderful work that you are doing for yourself and your family.

Review Of Topics Covered

- The importance of assessing clutter.
- How to begin your assessment.
- Things to observe on your assessment walk.

Visualization For Chapter 7
Assess For Success

Sit down in an uncluttered area of your home. Create a quiet space by closing the door or turning off the ringer on your phone(s). Take three cleansing breaths in through your nose and out the mouth. Close your eyes and imagine that you have invited an interior decorator to your home to discuss with you the changes you want to make.

You feel a little ashamed about the condition of your home. All your stuff will be exposed to her scrutiny. You know that your home represents who you are and who you wish to become. So, what does your space say about you? You tap into your feelings and use your intuition as you have been taught. Ah, yes, you feel it now. Your self-esteem and energy have decreased and there are some things that give you an uncomfortable feeling.

As you walk into each room with the decorator, you become aware that she is not interested in your messes. She is only interested in what color(s), furniture, and design changes are on your list. As you follow her, you see your home with new eyes.

You ask yourself, "Do I **love** everything I see, and do I want a relationship with it?" Yes, it's that simple. In former chapters you learned of the interconnectedness of everything. You have decided that you want your space to reflect who you really are and have decided to make some plans for future projects to accomplish this.

As you say goodbye to the decorator, you realize how much you have learned from this walk. Assessing all your worldly possessions does not seem as daunting a task as it did before, and you are now using your intuition easily.

Open your eyes and know that you can handle your clutter because you are setting goals and will break each project down into manageable tasks.

Journaling Ideas

- What are the results of your assessment walk?
- How do you feel about the most pressing areas?
- List some ways you can use your intuition.
- List some ways that you can become more aware of your intuition and your feelings.
- List your short-term and long-term goals.

Chapter 8

Starting on Your First Project(s)

Dear Lord: So far today, I am doing all right. I have not gossiped, lost my temper, been greedy, hasty, selfish, or self-indulgent. I have not whined, bitched, cursed, or eaten any chocolate. I have not charged on my credit card. However, I am going to get out of bed in a few minutes, and I will need a lot more help after that. Amen.

—Author Unknown

There comes a time in our lives when we say, "**Enough! I have to do something about this state of affairs!**"

Taking control of your clutter enables you to live in the present and manage your life with more assurance and ease. You can clear the cobwebs and enter a space where you have control over your life and feel good about yourself. You will actively begin to work on your clutter.

Unless you have decided to call a junk dealer, you can use some boxes. Your local supermarket will always have some for you. Pick up at least five for starters. You may need more later.

Possible Labels For Boxes

- Trash/Recycle
- Donate/Charity
- Garage Sale
- Transition
- Repairs

As you go over the piles, drawers, closets, etc., you will sort clutter into the various boxes. You may find my labels don't work for you. Please create ones that do. When you are done with an area or a pile that you have designated as your goal for the session, take each box to a place where you can store it until the items contained in it are taken care of. For instance:

Trash/Recycling can be bagged and put out with the garbage.

Donations/Charity can be put in the car to deliver to your favorite thrift store or charity when you are running errands.

Repairs can also go in the car.

The **Transition** box might need to be the biggest one. Put a note on your calendar to check its contents in one, three, or six months. Before you open it, try to remember what's in it. Your life has gone on well without all those things. Did you miss or need any of them? Now you can give yourself permission to either sell, give away, or recycle any or all of those items. Any designated as keepers can be put away in their appropriate places.

> **Important:** Don't create piles from your cleaning with the intention of going through them at a later date. Make your decisions as you do your work. You may begin to feel a lot of resistance because you are trying to get rid of stuff to which you are attached.

Paper Clutter

Make a promise to follow each piece of paper to its logical and rightful place. Give each piece of paper a home. If you don't have a file for that particular subject, either make one or put the paper in a file labeled **To Be Decided**. Clip those articles from newspapers and magazines that you would like to read and put them in a special file labeled **To Read**. Recycle the newspapers and magazines that remain. Piles of unread newspapers and magazines collect dust, remind you of all the things you have to do, and provide fuel for the fires of procrastination.

Think of your files as extensions of your mind. They are there to help you organize your thoughts and activities and build order and focus in your life.

Use sub-categories in your filing system to separate bank statements from credit card statements, for an example.

Reserve your desktop for items used on a daily basis. Make good use of wall space for multi-tiered organizers.

Several of the books in the resource guide have excellent chapters on how to deal with papers, mail, and files. Your local library can get them from Inter-Library Loan if they don't have them.

Organize Your Home, Ronni Eisenberg and Kate Kelly
Lighten Up, Michelle Passoff
The New Messies Manual, Sandra Felton
Organizing From The Inside Out, Julie Morgenstern
Getting Organized, Stephanie Winston

Mail Clutter

You pick up your mail everyday, then it becomes a problem. Why? Every piece of mail requires a home immediately, or it will end up entangled with other bits of paper and disappear in the general mountain of papers that grows daily all by itself.

Choose to give each piece of mail a home. I leave my junk mail unopened, recycle it, and read only those pieces that either interest or are of importance to me. This eliminates a great deal of clutter from entering the house.

Bills, correspondence, or important documents need to be put in their designated places as soon as possible, if not immediately. Bills can be filed away as you pay them. Mark them paid and note the date. I personally use two huge plastic clothes pins that someone gave me to hold bills and important papers. You can purchase bulldog clips or use file folders for each category. If you have extra drawers, they can be put there. Baskets are attractive and cheap. You can hang them on a peg system that is designed for coats. Check the resource guide.

Place catalogs, magazines, and newspapers in a special basket or holder until you get to them. I have a large, sturdy, 4" deep basket at the end of my desk for odds and ends of paper that accumulate weekly from various sources. They pile up for several weeks to a month then I file or recycle them. While they are waiting for me, they are kept safe and neat.

Clothing Clutter

It is important to look at all the clothes in your closet and commit yourself to being firm and, if necessary, severe. Ask yourself the following questions:

- Does it fit?
- Is it in season?
- Is it clean, pressed, and mended?
- Does it fit my present lifestyle?
- Will I really wear it?

Look inside again with these other criteria in mind:

- Recognize that we wear only 20% of our clothes 80% of the time. It is the clothes we rarely wear that take up the space.
- Clear out all empty hangars and store them in one section of the closet.
- All hangars should be of the same type.
- Hang like things with like things.
- Put similar colors together within each clothing category.
- Clear out all clothes that are not in season. Store these elsewhere, perhaps in the back of the closet, or create a closet just for out-of-season items.
- Clear out all clothes that you haven't worn in a year or two for whatever reason. Your fat and skinny clothes can be stored separately or in the back of the closet.

Patty Heller, a student of mine, shared these wonderful ideas:

- Ask yourself if the new 'me' wants what is in the closet. You may have changed so much that a change is called for in your clothing selection.
- Prepare a new wardrobe for that person. You can do this in stages and can start frequenting thrift stores for good buys.
- Look at your colors; they may be changing as you change.
- Too many choices in your closet? An over-stuffed closet can create blockages and pull your energy down.

It is also a good idea to have a light in your closet. You can purchase a battery-powered type that does not need an electrician to install. It is wonderful when you can see everything in your closet.

You will see a big difference in the belts, ties, and scarves situation when you install an attractive holder for these items.

Use a clear plastic shoe bag on the inside of hall closets. Store adult stuff in the highest pockets and kids stuff in the lowest.

Book Clutter

Many people derive a sense of pleasure and a measure of security from looking at their book collections. They like to look at their bookcases filled with books they have never read but like to have there just in case.

Several years ago I went through all my books, and there were a lot. I remembered back to the days when I never gave any thought to my purchases. Now I evaluate the book I am interested in, write down its name and author, and go to the Library to have them get it for me if it's not on their shelves. If I think it's a keeper, I buy it. I am so happy to have put the old pattern behind me.

I decided that I wasn't going to keep any book that I hadn't used for two years. I kept a few I was certain would be useful, even though I hadn't used them recently. It felt so good to sell hundreds of books that I carted around with me to all the places I had lived in the last fifteen years. Now I had some cash and in the process discovered that I didn't miss one of them. You can make a list of some books that you are very attached to and can get them from the library or donate them to the library and take them out whenever you desire.

I am a weaver and, in 1999, decided to go over my extensive collection of weaving and craft books. I was totally honest with myself in looking at each and every book in my collection. I gave some to my weaving guild library, others were set aside for our guild auction, some were sold, and the rest were given to charity. I had some duplicates, some contained material that I would never use in twenty lifetimes, and others were just not of interest to me anymore. It felt so good, so freeing. Now I only have those books that serve me, interest me, or have reference value.

Books are highly replaceable. Books are wonderful, I admit. They can also become a drag on your life. You have to dust them, move them when you do, and they can also serve as a reminder of all the things and ideas that you wanted to pursue but never did (shades of procrastination popping up). By clearing your books you provide space for new ideas to take hold and for the winds of change and opportunity to enter your life.

Children And Clutter

Households with children and lots of different schedules to track, as well as homework assignments, appointments, and messages, are beset with clutter on an ongoing basis. The kitchen is often the center of it, and mostly that's where the master calendar and message boards are hung. It's also where everyone tends to "hang out," going to the fridge, making phone calls, etc. Here are some helpful hints for you.

- Divide a bulletin board into sections or quadrants by category or by child. Appointments, important phone numbers, shopping needs, reminders, activities, things that come due at a certain date are categories to consider. Look over the bulletin board and also the door of the fridge weekly and recycle anything outdated.
- File away the children's drawings, photos, projects, or assignments that merit preserving in a box for each child or in an appropriate container.

- Keep an **IN** box or folder for each child to hold his or her mail, permission slips, graded papers, report cards, and projects. Go over their stuff with them often and take pictures of things that are too big to keep. Decide with your child what are keepers from the rest.

- Keep a section of the board for notes and messages with a pen close by. You can buy boards that are divided into bulletin and writing areas in office supply stores for $12-$20.

- Look for clear plastic hanging organizers or shoe bags that can fit over doorways or in closets. They are great for kids' stuff, cosmetics, sundries, etc. There are some products like this in Lillian Vernon's catalog for storage ideas.

- Purchase mini chests on wheels for the corners near where your children do their homework and art projects and for storage of odds and ends. They can also be used as a recycling center. Those units with three-five clear plastic drawers are $20 at Office Max; Bed, Bath, and Beyond; Lowe's; and K-Mart. Try Target, Pier One, and the catalogs in the resource guide for other choices.

Here are some tips from an article in *Family Circle* 9/1/97 that can help you with children's clutter. "Closet Cleanup" by Stephanie Denton suggests that you take the kids when you donate items. It teaches them generosity, empathy, and gets across the idea that you are engaged in the whole clutter cleaning "thing." Your example will teach them a lot. Let your children pick out, decorate, and label their own storage containers. And lastly, remember that for any system to work, convenience is the key.

We have worked on creating order and organization in this chapter. Stephanie Winston says, "Order is not an end in itself. It is what helps you function effectively and effortlessly in your space." She describes order as:

- A physical environment that is easy to move around in.
- An environment that is easy to look at.
- An environment that is easy to function in.
- An environment that provides a simple and effective way to deal with paperwork, mail, filing, etc.

She also presents "the organizing principle." Use flexible thinking and analyze your alternatives. Good advice to follow — especially when confronted with endless decisions and so many new ideas.

Review Of Topics Covered

- Preparing boxes for sorting.
- Cleaning paper, mail, books, clothing, and children's clutter.
- Definition of order.

Visualization For Chapter 8
Living Lean

Sit down in an uncluttered area of your home. Create a quiet space by closing the door or turning off the ringer on your phone(s). Take three cleansing breaths in through your nose and out the mouth. Close your eyes and imagine that you are visiting your child's nursery school for a special event. The teachers are going to take you on a tour and describe how the rooms are organized.

The first thing you see is a very neat and orderly room that is divided into areas of activity: music, arts and crafts, reading, dress-up, eating, and clean-up. In each there are attractive boxes and cubbies with labels on them. Some of the containers are colored, and you are told that this has a purpose. Color coding is used extensively in organizing. The children are aware of what each color stands for.

You realize that you feel comfortable and at ease knowing where everything goes. This simplifies life. You resolve to create some aspects of this order in your own home. Creating a place for each thing, labeling boxes and shelves, and putting things back where they belong are high on your priority list.

There is a spareness and neatness to the space that makes you feel supported and nurtured. You understand how children can learn in such a environment, how they can find fun things to do, and how it teaches them good skills for life.

You smile to yourself as you remember reading Lao Tzu's idea that knowledge and peace are acquired as you let go of something everyday. You promise yourself that you will begin to practice this and those things that you learned at the nursery school.

Open your eyes and feel pleased with what you have accomplished.

Journaling Ideas

- Create your own categories for your sorting boxes.
- List things you can do to create more order in your paper, mail, book, clothing, and children's clutter.
- List the things that would create more order in your life.

Chapter 9

Staying Clutter Free From Now On

*In the pursuit of knowledge, everyday
something is added. In the pursuit of the Tao,
everyday something is dropped.*

—Lao Tzu

You will discover as you clean the clutter in your physical environment that movement will automatically occur in your mental, emotional, and spiritual realms as well. Everything is interconnected. Be prepared for the unexpected and unpredictable as you lift the dust and debris of years of chaotic thinking, living, and feeling. My students have reported this, other authors have written about it, and **Feng Shui** guarantees it. Things will settle down as you start to practice the suggestions in this book When your stuff is organized, put where it belongs, and kept that way, you will feel a great sense of balance and harmony in your life. Read on to find out ways to keep this feeling going.

AN INTRODUCTION TO A CLUTTER-FREE LIFE

It is important to learn to say no to buying and become determined to eliminate items that are no longer serving or nurturing you.

Recycling is an important option to consider instead of throwing away things that will become part of the general landfill. There are always people who can use what you no longer can. Think of charities, a garage sale, thrift shops, and friends and relations as sources for gifting things you no longer desire to have around you.

As your home becomes more clutter free and organized, your life will change accordingly, and it will be easier to keep it that way in the future.

Breaking each task down into small portions or jobs that can be done in the time you have scheduled will be of great assistance to you.

Following is a list that will guide you in ways to remain clutter free. Think about them, then decide how you are going to institute them into your daily life. Perhaps do three a week. It is also important to discuss them with others who live with you.

Staying Clutter Free

- Store like things with like things.
- Keep things near to where they are used.
- Make it easy to put things where they belong.
- Assign everything in your home a designated place.
- Put things you use the most in the easiest places to get to; like the front of the drawer or shelf.

- Ban "for nows" and get in the habit of putting stuff in its place right away. Take things upstairs each time you go there.
- If you bring something new in, resolve that something has to go.
- Do clutter cleaning on a regular basis instead of letting things get out of hand.
- Think twice before you buy. Don't go shopping for entertainment, go with a purpose in mind.
- Establish a junk drawer for each member of the household and clean them out regularly.
- Buy yourself a labeler at an office supply store. They make very attractive and sturdy labels for all your things.
- Try to put purchases away as soon as you can.
- Don't add to a pile or area that you are working on.
- Stick with your project until you have finished it. Watch out for distractions.
- Look ahead for the benefits you will derive from a clutter-free environment.
- Reward yourself frequently for staying clutter free.

Maintaining a Clutter-Free Desk and Office

- Give every item in your home/office a designated place.
- Maintain a clear desktop.
- Look for attractive baskets and clear plastic containers to store desk stuff and other odds and ends.
- Label them clearly.
- Avoid information overload. You can't read everything or save everything — be selective.
- Work from files, not from piles. File papers as soon as you can. Buy a filing cabinet if you don't already have one. You can find these in resale shops and discount or used office supply stores.

- Reward yourself frequently.
- Bring professionals and others in to help you when you need their service because of a time crunch or skill needed for the job.
- Keep a log or notebook by the phone for calls that are received and check them off when you answer them. This will also become an invaluable source of information.
- Keep notes on projects and to-do lists in another notebook.
- Learn to rely on to-do lists. Plan your day and try to get accomplished what you can. Don't be hard on yourself if you don't. There's always tomorrow.

Attention to Details

The following suggestions are reminders to help you stay focused on making clutter-clearing habits a part of your everyday life.

- Straighten up your kitchen and living room (or where you spend your evenings) before going to bed. This will make you feel organized and complete for the day, ensuring you a restful night's sleep.
- Make use of odd bits of time to do chores such as mail sorting, folding clothes, answering phone calls, writing letters, paying bills, and writing your shopping and to-do lists.
- These bits of time arrive when you are watching the news, during commercials, while you are waiting for dinner to cook, while doing the dishes, while the kids are doing their homework, or while waiting in your car for someone.

Bed-Making Technique

This method offers you a very quick and easy way to make your bed every morning. Doing this helps you start the day with order and also gives you a neat bed to slide into as the day ends.

- Put your bottom sheet on the mattress
- Spread a cover sheet over this, then put your quilt or blankets over this.
- Tuck in the cover sheet and quilt/blankets at the foot of the bed (and, if desired, 1/4 of the way up the sides as well).
- Smooth the cover sheet and pull the headboard edge over a little to cover quilts or blankets at their top edge.
- Spread your bedspread or comforter over this if you use one and arrange your pillows.

Every morning:

- **Straighten the bottom sheet.**
- **Pull the cover sheet up. Fold its edge over your quilt or blanket.**
- **Pull all tight.**
- **Finish with spreading your top cover over all.**
- **Place your pillows as desired.**

These steps take one to two minutes and often can be done with going around the bed only once. The secret is tucking in the edges of your cover sheet and quilt. This tends to keep everything neat and allows you to make your bed quickly in the morning.

Straightening up before retiring and making the bed first thing in the morning are examples of bringing order to your life and creating patterns of discipline that work to eliminate clutter.

I am including the following list to help you with the very important issues of mental and emotional clutter. Think about them, then decide which ones you can start to work on now. Perhaps do three a week, then assess how they have made a difference in your life.

Staying Free of Mental and Emotional Clutter

- Stop worrying, criticizing, judging, and blaming (self or others).
- Be clear in your communications with yourself and others.
- Keep up to date with your correspondence and returning phone calls.
- Decide to work on your unresolved issues if they haven't cleared up with clutter cleaning.
- Don't watch the news or anything violent on TV before retiring. The stations know that the news is depressing or violent, so they have been ending on a high note or with something humorous.
- Stay focused on what you set out to do. Avoid distracting yourself with "grasshopper" type work habits (that is, jumping from one project or area of the house to another before completing what you started).
- Live in the present moment by keeping things up to date.
- Let go of old grievances, resentments, and bitterness.
- Watch out for any emotional armoring that might surface.
- Let go of old ways of reacting. This includes whining and complaining.
- Move on in relationships that don't nurture you.
- Forgive yourself and move on.
- Honor your time to do clutter cleaning as a way of honoring yourself.
- Scattered thinking can become a thing of the past if you start to meditate.
- Creating dramas and reacting to criticism or imagined slights can also be helped with meditating on a regular basis.
- Use the **chi** lifters in Chapter 6 to reduce stress, anxiety, worry, and tension.

New Ways of Looking at Old Ideas

Honor yourself and change your outlook at the same time!

• • •

Housework is really the privilege
of managing your home.
Cleaning your room is actually treating
yourself with dignity.
Organizing and filing becomes relieving
the stress of chaos.
Keeping things picked up is embracing
harmony in your life.
Making the kids keep things organized is training
them for responsible adulthood.

— Sandra Felton

• • •

"Act as if you already embody you goal," remarks Suze
Orman in *The Courage To Be Rich*. Why not start doing this
right now? It is such an empowering thought. You can start
by doing the visualizations at the end of each chapter. They will
help to incorporate into your life the symbols that influence you
for the better. You can practice your goals in these visualizations which will bring you one step closer to doing them.

After I graduated from Massage School, it was hard for me
to believe that I was a Massage Therapist. I bought a massage
table and all the necessaries to work with. I had cards printed
and started to spread the word that I was open for business. I
was acting as if I embodied my goal, and it worked. I began to
have more confidence in myself and started to attract clients.

We are now ready to embark on our **Feng Shui** adventure.
Read on to find out ways to incorporate this 3,000-year-old
body of wisdom into clutter cleaning projects.

Review of Topics Covered

- How to stay clutter free.
- How to maintain a clutter-free desk and office.
- Some details of clutter-free living.
- How to stay free of mental and emotional clutter.
- Acting as if you embody your goal.

Visualization for Chapter 9
The Real You

Sit down in an uncluttered area of your home. Create a quiet space by closing the door or turning off the ringer on your phone(s). Take three cleansing breaths in through your nose and out the mouth. Close your eyes and imagine going through your first project of clutter cleaning with ease. You prepare well and do the small jobs first, gaining a feeling of success as you progress to the more difficult and involved ones. You are practicing your goal by visualizing it first.

Diving into papers, piles, books, and, yes, into your closets — that last bastion of walled-off clutter. You are poised in front of your clothes. Imagine the new you emerging from all this with clothes and possessions that express who you really are.

You smile to yourself as you remember the chaos that reigned just a few weeks ago. You now view your domain with calm and focus. You've come a long way, baby.

As order has become more of a daily habit rather than a wish, you are able to be so much more authentic and honest with yourself and in all your communications. Scattered and unfocused thinking is beginning to be a thing of the past. Nurturing and supporting all aspects of yourself and practicing the suggestions about language, **shoulding**, and saying **no** have given you the courage to speak with your heart, not with your mind all the time. It has changed the flavor of your messages to yourself because, after all, you hear and feel the words you are saying as well as your audience.

Now the possibility exists that you can accept yourself as a powerful being worthy of respect and honor and not pushing parts of yourself aside and denying parts of yourself.

Open your eyes and know that this new you is the real you and feel wonderful about all that you have achieved.

Journaling Ideas

- List some things you can do to stay clutter free.
- List some things you can do to relieve emotional and mental clutter.
- List some things you can do to "act as if you embody your goal."

_____

_____

_____

_____

_____

_____

_____

_____

_____

_____

_____

_____

Chapter 10

Using Feng Shui and the Bagua

First we shape our dwellings, then our dwellings shape us.

—Winston Churchill

How can **Feng Shui** and the **Bagua** (pronounced bahg-wa) help with our clutter cleaning projects? **Feng Shui** acknowledges with compassion the difficulties which arise from living. It views the world and all things in it (humans, animals, rocks, water, vegetation, planets, stars, and all man-made objects) as involved in a dynamic relationship where each thing affects the other. **Feng Shui** incorporates the following fields of knowledge: intuition, spirituality, interior design, psychology, folk wisdom, symbology, flow of **chi**, color, and good common sense. The marrying of all these with 3,000 years of accumulated wisdom from many cultures creates a system that can affect you on many levels and change your life for the better. You have discovered how to use this knowledge in the preceding chapters.

The **Feng Shui** ideas I have introduced to you include the concept that cluttered thoughts create physical clutter and that physical clutter creates confused and disorganized thinking. This occurs because of the interconnection of all things and the ability of **chi** to influence you, your environment, and your possessions.

The Bagua

The **Bagua** is an ancient Chinese symbol and tool for explaining life's paths and pitfalls. It is composed of nine sections and is an octagon, which is a sacred symbol to the Chinese and many of the cultures in the Orient. It is a wonderful tool that describes aspects of your life and places these in a template covering your home which then enables you to work on your life issues. This map, template, or mandala helps you focus on and become aware of these issues or problems.

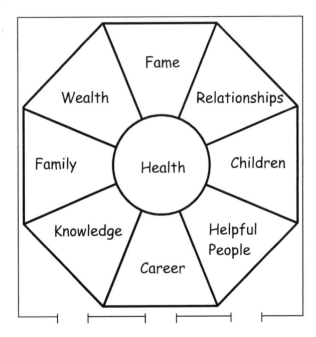

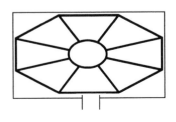

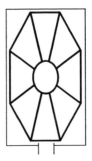

The size of the square **Bagua** can expand or decrease to fit the dimensions of your floorplan/home.

Following is a diagram of the **Bagua** simplified into a square so that you can easily superimpose it onto the floorplan of your home. If you discover that your home has missing areas, instructions can be found in many **Feng Shui** books that will help you with this problem. You may also want to consult these books to increase your knowledge of **Feng Shui**. This manual is not intended to cover **Feng Shui** completely; just enough to help you use the information for clutter cleaning purposes. The square **Bagua** looks like this:

Prosperity Wealth Fortunate Blessings Abundance	Fame Reputation Success Recognition	Relationships Love Marriage Friends
Family Elders Community Ancestors	Center Unity Health	Creativity Children Projects Future
Knowledge Skills Wisdom Self-Improvement	Career Path in Life Journey	Helpful People Benefactors Travel

FRONT OF HOUSE — THE BAGUA

The first step is to determine where your front door falls in the **Bagua**. Notice that there are three possible entrances: **Knowledge**, **Career**, and **Helpful People**. Most front doors fall into one of these. If yours does not, or you use another door as your main door, you can examine each room in the house separately.

Stand in the doorway of the room and decide what entrance it corresponds to (**Knowledge**, **Career**, **Helpful People**). If the doorway is in the center of the room, then it is in the **Career** area. If it is to the left, it is in the **Knowledge** area, and if it is to the right, it is in the **Helpful People** area. You can now orient yourself because each room is being used as a separate and complete **Bagua**.

In applying the **Bagua** to your home, you will draw a floorplan of your home. You can then divide your floorplan into the nine sections as illustrated and use it to find what rooms in your home correspond to each sector of the **Bagua**.

It is now time for you to take a look at your home. Hold the square **Bagua** in front of you and see where the rooms in your floorplan mesh with the nine sections of the **Bagua**. Turn your drawing until the front of your house is parallel to the lower edge of the **Bagua**.

You will now apply the **Bagua** and its descriptions of life areas to your home. If you have a second floor or a lower level in your home, apply the **Bagua** in the same way to those areas.

What did you find out? Is your bedroom in the **Relationships** section of the **Bagua,** or is it in the **Wealth** section? Do this with each room. Where is the most clutter in your home, or are there pockets in certain areas? You now have more knowledge to assess your home on even deeper levels.

Note the rooms, their condition, and what life descriptions appear. Are they filled with clutter, is the artwork sad, is the placement of furniture not encouraging good flow of **chi**? Looking at the descriptions of each life area as they apply to the rooms in your home/workplace can help you determine which ones need work and how to bring about positive change. Please refer to the questions, listing of important life areas, the addtional words, and **Feng Shui** hints for assistance in finding where to work, how to work, and what to apply to the sector of the **Bagua** that you desire to enhance.

Go to the area under your kitchen sink where there are many "miracle" cleaners waiting to be used. You find they are crammed in along with lots of other stuff. You don't even remember what's in there. Using the theory of symbols these may represent all the parts of you that you are not in touch with or want to recognize. Look at your plan and see what section of the **Bagua** it falls into. In each section, the descriptions identify what specific human experiences flourish there.

Let's suppose your kitchen is in the **Family** section. Peer into your life. Do you feel some block regarding family or authority issues? The messy and stuffed space housing your cleaners creates blocks to free-flowing **chi**. Some additional ideas for reflection are past history, place among others, as well as the amount of discipline in your life.

Looking at the symbology of the physical items in a room gives you a new way to view the descriptions of life experiences in the **Bagua**. Doing a clean-out of the area could bring you clarity, security, discipline, and easier relationships with family and authority.

You can now look at each room of your home/workplace to find out more about yourself, clean the clutter there, and discover how this can clear up the issues. I have designed the following "Questions to Ponder," "Important Life Areas," and "Additional Descriptions for the Bagua" as ways to help you do this.

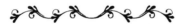

In applying the principles outlined in this chapter, you will examine all your things and your thought processes. This helps to bring more love into your life. Carol Bridges, in *The Medicine Woman's Guide to Being in Business for Yourself*, says, "You have demonstrated the power to gather love to yourself by gathering the things you love and taking care of them. . . . You have experienced the exquisite emptiness of holding onto nothing unloved."

QUESTIONS TO PONDER

- What is the room(s) where clutter is most evident?
- What part of the **Bagua** is that room in?
- What kinds of things are there, what kind of clutter, and how much?
- What is the level of organization or disorganization in the room or pile?
- What is the area of your life that needs attention the most? Is that the area that has the most clutter or disorganization?
- What is the area of the **Bagua** or the room that you have chosen to work on? This might be your most urgent or frustrating problem?
- When you look at the **Bagua** and note the rooms with the most problem areas, also look at the descriptions that go with that space and see if these have any meaning for you. They could suggest emotions, relationships that need work, activities that need adjusting, and goals that need attention.
- What are your possessions saying to you? How do they make you feel? This is using your intuition.

The following information is designed to help you assess each section of the **Bagua** as it applies to your home/ workplace. It is condensed and therefore is not as complete as you will find when you explore other books on **Feng Shui**. This is meant as a start to look at the topics of abundance, health, career, relationships, etc.

Important Life Areas

PROSPERITY-WEALTH-FORTUNATE BLESSINGS-ABUNDANCE

Consider how you create and maintain wealth and attract all forms of abundance. Clutter here can cause blocks to cash flow and create roadblocks of all kinds.

FAME-REPUTATION-SUCCESS-RECOGNITION

How do you acquire your fame and reputation? Clutter in this area can dampen and dull your popularity, passion, and enthusiasm and create problems relating to finalizing projects.

RELATIONSHIPS-LOVE-MARRIAGE FRIENDS-CLIENTS

What is the quality of all your relationships? Clutter can cause difficulty in finding a mate or satisfying links with other people.

CREATIVITY-CHILDREN-PROJECTS-FUTURE

Are you pleased with the level of creative ideas in your life, do projects go smoothly, and are your children thriving and happy? Clutter can cause struggle to appear in these areas.

HELPFUL PEOPLE-BENEFACTORS-TRAVEL

Are you attracting help of all kinds into your life in the amounts that you desire? Clutter in this area can create obstacles to the flow of support and movement in your life and work.

CAREER-PATH IN LIFE-LIFE JOURNEY

Is your career fulfilling and are you pleased with the path you are following in life? Clutter can cause life to feel like a struggle and create fogginess about your goals.

KNOWLEDGE-SKILLS-WISDOM SELF-IMPROVEMENT

Are you growing through increased self-knowledge? Clutter can cause limitations in your ability to make decisions and follow through with plans.

FAMILY-ELDERS-COMMUNITY-ANCESTORS

Do you have satisfying relationships with family, parents, and community. Clutter can cause difficulties with persons in authority, parents, and the amount of discipline in your life.

CENTER-UNITY-HEALTH

Consider if you have a sense of purpose and balance in your life. Clutter can cause a breakdown in aspects of your overall health as well as limit your ability to concentrate. (In many homes the center is empty, and we walk through this area to get to other areas. Therefore you can apply **Health** to the **Family** area.)

The words in the following summary offer you more suggestions to look at life descriptions in the **Bagua**. Apply them to your life, work, and goals to determine if you have these in the amounts that you desire or if clutter in these zones block them from being a part of your life/work.

ADDITIONAL DESCRIPTIONS FOR THE BAGUA

Wealth — Empowerment, opportunity, resources, needs met, freedom from limits, and orderliness.

Fame — Achievements, honoring self, and self-expression.

Relationships — Intimacy, sharing of self, and commitment.

Creativity — Playfulness and being grounded.

Helpful People — Nurturing and support from others and networking.

Career — Life purpose, goals, and self-appreciation.

Knowledge — Dreams, self-discovery, and spiritual growth.

Family — Roots, past history, tradition, and your place among others.

Health — Nourishment of body and soul.

FENG SHUI HINTS FOR EACH ROOM

I include the following **Feng Shui** hints for creating more balance and harmony in your home.

The Bedroom — Comfy, cozy, serene, sensual, and restful. If there is clutter here, the flow of renewing and beneficial **chi** could decrease. Can you see the door from your bed? Use items in pairs to improve the possibility and quality of relationships.

The Bathroom — Neat and upward moving. The overall energy here is damp, moist, and draining. Clear counters to encourage movement of **chi**. Plants and floral wallpaper can help increase the element of upward growth and vitality to counter the influence of so many drains.

The Kitchen — Where physical nourishment is stored and prepared. Stress can be reduced if order and cleanliness are maintained. A mirror behind the stove can alleviate any anxiety the cook might experience if he/she can't see who is entering the room while cooking.

The Dining Room — Free of clutter. Eating can become a beautiful and social ritual that encourages ease of digestion and communication between family members.

The Living Room, Den, or Family Room — Where we get ideas and knowledge, and have fun. Encourage ease of movement and conversation so that relationships are enhanced and relaxation is easy. One focal point is good.

Front Door, Entrance, Front Hall—Free of clutter and "en-trancing." Look behind doors; they need to open fully (symbol of allowing opportunity to enter and **chi** to flow freely). A **Feng Shui** custom of taking shoes off before entering the home can keep the energy of the outside world out to make your home a sanctuary. It is what impacts you and your guests first and is remembered. Create a pleasant ambiance and lots of plants to look at before you get to the door. This will help you leave the tensions of the day behind and lift your spirits. Your front door represents who you are and who you wish to become (as indeed your whole house does).

> **Important: Adjusting things in your space by looking at them as symbols that influence how you feel can truly heal and transform.**

I had a client who wanted a relationship. There was a lot of clutter in her bedroom, and she never made the bed. After clearing the clutter, making the bed every day (preparing for company), putting pairs of things around the room and on the bed, an old boyfriend called and a relationship restarted.

This is the kind of success that I wish for you.

Turn to the next chapter to find out neat facts that other authors have for you on clutter. This chapter is very important, so don't overlook it.

Review of Topics Covered

- Description of the **Bagua**.
- Questions to ask as you look at your floorplan.
- Hints for creating more harmony in your home.

Visualization for Chapter 10
Finding Courage

Sit down in an uncluttered area of your home. Create a quiet space by closing the door or turning off the ringer on your phone(s). Take three cleansing breaths in through your nose and out the mouth. Imagine the **Bagua** in your mind. Picture your floorplan superimposed over it.

You have not had the courage to start using this diagram, but you know that **Feng Shui** has achieved great results for many people, so you decide to give it a try.

You decide to look into the spare bedroom which is in the **Creativity**, **Children**, and **Projects** area of life. How fortunate, you won't have to disturb anyone's decor for your project. Look around the room. Are there any areas that could use cleaning? You have made the connection that any piles of clutter here could be hampering projects that you want to start.

Gathering up all the supplies you need to complete the job will make things go even faster than you expected. Somehow all aspects of this enterprise fall into place and you are able to plan how to finish

Cleaning the clutter in this room does not take too long. You feel a lot better. You know you can work on the projects you have put off for so long. You find yourself working with focus and renewed energy. The room somehow feels lighter, brighter, and easier to move around in it. You realize there is a connection between cleaning clutter and freeing up energy that blocked you from working on your projects.

You smile to yourself and know that great amounts of energy will be released with each project that gets completed and with that more courage to do others.

Open your eyes feeling happy, filled with courage, and relieved to know that these methods really do work

Journaling Ideas

- List areas of your life that you want to work on using the words in the sections of the **Bagua**.
- List three things your possessions are saying to you.
- List three areas of your home that need attention because they have clutter there.

_____

_____

_____

_____

_____

_____

_____

_____

_____

_____

_____

_____

_____

_____

_____

_____

_____

Chapter 11

Gems from the Minds

*When you undervalue what you do, the world
will undervalue who you are.*

— Suze Orman, *The Courage To Be Rich*

Sifting through all this data was actually a very pleasant
task and fruitful for my purposes of gathering knowledge from
allied fields that broaden the scope of clutter cleaning.

Many of the authors and professionals agree on particular
issues, while they emphasize certain specific areas in their
books. Knowing that you have limited amounts of time, I have
endeavored to present help for you from different sources,
while including ideas that will provide ways to effect the
changes you want.

Most of the information in this chapter does not appear
elsewhere in the book. Naturally, I would not want to be
responsible for adding to your book clutter, so I recommend
borrowing them first before buying. If, however, you are in a
bookstore and one speaks to you, by all means buy it. Just get
rid of one book to keep the balance going.

Books and Authors

Organizing From The Inside Out, by Julie Morgenstern

This book has been on the *Times* Best-seller List. In Chapters 6-9 of Part 3 are ways to clean closets. Pages 127-133 list ways to sort, label, and store papers, bills, and documents. There is also a good chapter on the home office. Ms. Morgenstern has some other great ideas as well:

- ~ You hold all your successes inside of you as well as all the former you's and don't need to keep the papers or memorabilia.
- ~ There is no good or bad; don't judge yourself.
- ~ Professional cleaners say that getting rid of excess clutter reduces housework by 40%.
- ~ For a messy mate, provide a basket for all the stuff thrown on the floor.
- ~ Research says that the average American spends one hour a day looking for stuff and one hour procrastinating. That equals six weeks a year for each.
- ~ Adopt a charity to give your stuff to and feel good about yourself.
- ~ Use the kindergarten method of having a place for everything: labeled containers and similar things grouped and stored together, sometimes according to activities.

Clutter's Last Stand and Clutter Free, by Don Aslett

Mr. Aslett presents some very practical advice in a very humorous format. His books are easy to read and to the point. He has many other titles.

- ~ Clutter makes every job take longer.
- ~ Are you paying $300 a year to store $150 worth of stuff in a rental unit?

~ Look at your relationships. Are they filled with clutter, too?

~ Beware of TV offers and gadget buying.

~ Start your clutter cleaning with easy projects such as under the kitchen sink, linen closet, purse, car, medicine cabinet, jewelry, photos, spices, magazines, tapes or videos.

The Courage To Be Rich, by Suze Orman

This is an excellent book designed to help you with the clutter of your finances.

~ How many bank accounts do you have with just $25?

~ Release your hold over things that you have outgrown.

~ Keep your memories in your heart, not in your closet.

~ Don't let charm turn into chains.

~ People who are obsessive about clutter also overeat, overcook, overbuy, and overtalk.

Living The Simple Life, by Elaine St. James

This author has written several books about simplifying your life. They are all excellent. *Simplify Your Life, Simplify Your Christmas, Simplify Your Life With Kids, and Inner Simplicity.*

~ Opt for voluntary simplicity and midwife yourself. (What a great idea!)

~ Create a 30-day buying list. Think about the items, and if after 30 days you still desire them, buy them. Change your consumer mentality about Christmas buying and gift-giving. You will find that many people are ready to change this pattern, too, and only

need a go-ahead from you to signal a change; such as sending a handmade card or something simple to them.
~ Clear excess plants, tables, and pillows. We all have too many of these.

Organize Your Home, by Ronni Eisenberg and Kate Kelly, and *Organize Yourself*

This is a short but very packed book with information galore on every topic of clutter control and organization techniques for the home. Excellent chapter on how to handle your files.

> ~ Determine what is the purpose of every closet and stick to that.
> ~ Keep records of catalog orders and a running account of your contributions.

Getting Out From Under, by Stephanie Winston

This is her new book — every bit as good as *Getting Organized*.

> ~ There is a test to determine if you are a packrat.
> ~ There are superior chapters on downsizing, time management, reassessing your career and family issues.

Simply Organized, by Connie Cox and Cris Evatt

They have a good chapter on closets and clothes advising you to wear the clothes that you are ambivalent about and then make a decision about them. Their chapter on the home office is good.

> ~ They ask you to keep a carbon of every communication and also a record of everything you ask people to do. This is wise advice. Could also work with contracting work done on the home/workplace.

The New Messies Manual, by Sandra Felton

This is one of the best books I have read on this subject, and I highly recommend it for every area of clutter, organization, and more. Ms. Felton is the only author I know of who addresses the issue of ADD and Obsessive/ Compulsive Disorders. She has written books about these issues, as well as sponsoring support groups, a newsletter, and an organization that offers help. I thank her for teaching me that people who have these disorders have problems with clutter as part of their syndrome. See the resource guide for more information.

~ Cancel all magazine and newspapers that you don't read.

~ Simplify, sort, and store is the heart of organizing.

~ Write down your goals; this encourages stronger commitment.

~ When storing things in boxes in your garage, attic, or elsewhere, write on an index card what's in the box and tape it to the box. Also put this information on an another card for a file you keep on the boxes.

The Simple Life, by David Shi

A simply fascinating book about the history of living simply in this country.

~ Information about conspicuous consumption and the throw away mentality. He says the end result of this will bring about an energy crisis (that was in 1985). We are already there, aren't we?

~ Unbridled consumerism will foster a movement towards simpler living. (Hurray for Ralph Nader.)

~ Actually our country was founded by people who sought simplicity in life and living. It turns out this is an American ideal.

~ "The dynamo of advertising advanced capitalism which was on the verge of eliminating poverty altogether." Well that idea really went wrong somewhere. Advertising made people want more and this has led to a loss of self, community, and family, and has created a society of loners as well.

Clutter Control, by Jeff Campbell

His book, *Speed Cleaning*, has been recommended to me by many of my students. He has a unique way of showing you how much your clutter is costing you to keep. Take each room separately and measure zones of clutter length by width to get the square footage. Then multiply this figure by $1.00 per square foot. This amount represents how much you are paying each month to store, heat, cool, insure, and otherwise care for your stuff.

Lighten Up, by Michelle Passoff

~ She has a visualization process on pages 29-35 that is excellent.
~ Chapters on honoring time and creating a game plan are very helpful.
~ Chapters 6 & 7 on how to deal with paper are good.

The Medicine Woman's Guide to Being in Business for Yourself, by Carol Bridges

The subtitle tells all: How to Live by Your Spiritual Values in a Money-Based World. And that is exactly what is presented here, plus much more.

~ I especially liked the chapter on Healing.
~ Many unique and helpful activities are offered.

We have come to the end of this examination. There are so many wonderful books out there, and new ones come along all the time. Good luck to you in your search for just the right one(s).

Review of Topic Covered

- Books from authors that offer good material to use are listed, and points they make are included.

Visualization for Chapter 11
A Piece of the Pie

Sit down in an uncluttered area of your home. Create a quiet space by closing the door or turning off the ringer on your phone(s). Take three cleansing breaths in through your nose and out the mouth.

Let's take one book, one piece of the pie, and examine how to take the essence from it. *The New Messies Manual* by Sandra Felton comes to mind first. She presents many wonderful ideas that can be used easily.

Simplify, sort, and store is the heart of organizing, she says. What does simplify actually mean? Could you buy less, desire less, and organize your home so that everything has its own place (simplicity of space)? You think to yourself about all the ways that this can be done in your life. You will have to ask for help from your family or significant other(s).

What does sort mean? It means that you have to go over everything you own, once to weed out, then apply this principle every few months forever. Why? Because clutter forms constantly, and you have to keep at it or it can take over your life again.

What does store refer to? Give all things a designated spot. Accomplishing this will provide you with peace and calm in your life. Things may tend to lose their place. You know where they belong and will put them there so that order reigns. You now look at containers in a totally new way. They can be attractive, clear plastic, or baskets.

Order is a powerful thing; use it wisely.

You think to yourself what a terrific journey this has been. So much learned, so much accomplished, so much yet to do. You will do all that you desire and set goals for. You know that now. Procrastination is something you can deal with and change. Even though this habit has been around you for a long time, you now have the tools to deal with it.

Smiling to yourself, you see a rainbow that glows over your whole house/workplace/property giving you a sign that a new era has dawned in your life and productive changes are occurring.

Open your eyes and go about your day or evening with renewed vigor and enthusiasm to accomplish all that you wish for yourself and/or your family.

Journaling Ideas

- Review the books presented and decide which one(s) you desire to read.
- List three things that you learned from the books that were not presented anywhere else in this book.

_____

_____

_____

_____

_____

_____

_____

_____

_____

_____

_____

_____

_____

_____

_____

_____

_____

_____

_____

_____

_____

_____

_____

_____

_____

_____

_____

Chapter 12

The Gift

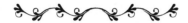

Today is a gift, that's why it's called the present.

—Author Unknown

Focusing on the present moment helps us achieve our goals. The past instructs, and the future can provide inspiration and dreams. Knowing how to use past, present, and future helps us become all that we can. Living in the present brings with it the desire and the necessity of addressing and solving problems that confront us. One of these is the clutter in our lives.

The issue of clutter is a multidimensional one composed of layers of feelings, thoughts, and experiences. A sense of powerlessness, anxiety, disorganization, and confusion occurs as piles and procrastination increase. Your self-esteem plummets as this happens on a daily basis. Self-esteem can begin to soar when you live in the present. Past events and experiences cease to intrude into your daily thoughts and life giving you hope and a positive outlook.

De-cluttering also helps restore self-esteem. It's a circle, isn't it? Poor self-esteem may be caused by clutter, and clutter can be the result of poor self-esteem.

"Everything you do is being in business for yourself," says Carol Bridges. Incorporating this idea into your life makes everything you do have value and honors you. Deciding on the merits of a purchase, rearranging a room, or cleaning a closet are all parts of being in business for yourself. This attitude elevates all your endeavors and increases self-esteem.

At the same time, it is wise to get professional help and read books that cover the subject of self-esteem. Meditation, visualization, and relaxation techniques will be of some assistance. Chapter 6 has many other suggestions for you as well.

Lack of self-esteem also spawns a random approach to life, which creates clutter. Random acts also create chaos. In the new physics, chaos is described as having order. This can be compared to the chaos that forms in our homes/workplaces. People keep doing the same things over and over again. Not putting papers away, not cleaning counters, or not being on time — there's an order to their chaos. I am not asking for ultra neatness and tidyness. That can become a problem, too. Some people who are very neat have hidden clutter. They put things behind doors and store stuff neatly. Too much stuff and things stored behind doors can limit opportunity and create energy blockages. Standing back and looking at yourself and your home/workplace with honesty and objectivity will provide more help. (See the quote about honesty at the end of this chapter.)

Honesty has many components, one of which is "Are you being/living consistent with your inner goals and desires?" Another is "Do your life and surroundings reflect who you really are and who you wish to become?" The quotes at the beginning of Chapters 1, 3, 5, and 6 and on the last page of this book contain messages about this topic. When you don't live your life in accord with your inner feelings, tension and anxiety mount, producing cluttering behaviors and material clutter that serve as a buffer screening out the lack of harmony in your life. These clutter-forming patterns sap your energy, control, and personal power. Restoring consistency between your inner and outer worlds and removing clutter from your environment and thoughts will return your energy, control, and personal power to you and elevate your self-esteem considerably.

Let us review the tools I have given you in this book. Keeping a journal of your journey to look back and see your progress and taking a step-by-step approach in planning projects and doing them for as little as ten minutes at a time, provided a start. Using **Feng Shui** to transform your environment and then influence changes in your physical, mental, emotional, and spiritual realms, while bringing more prosperity, better health and relationships, and more opportunity into your life was healing.

I have presented many diverse ideas to help you diminish the power clutter exerts on your life. In life, we do things together. With that in mind, I decided to include contributions other authors have made to the subject of clutter, organization, and living simply. The world of ideas is an interconnected one. An author's ideas have the power to create other solutions and even more ideas when read and tried. Since this book is about you, I searched for ways to make it as complete and as rich a source of help and information as I could

Good luck to you in everything that you wish to create for yourself. May all good things come to you. Walk forward into your journey with blessings. It has been such a great pleasure for me to present this book to you and help you create a better and more fulfilling life.

—Gaylah Balter, 2001

Review of Topics Covered

- A review of the sources of clutter
- Discussion of self-esteem and chaos.
- A review of methods to eliminate clutter.

Visualization for Chapter 12
Reviewing Your Day

I leave you with one last visualization. Each day before retiring, review your day. If any event was not harmonious or comfortable, recreate it in your mind and make it come out beneficial and nurturing for you. It is important to clear the day's events before going to sleep, especially if they have not been positive. We can learn from our experiences. I believe there are lessons for us in every event, every new experience, and interchange with people.

Journaling Ideas

- List ways you can improve your self-esteem.
- List ways you can eliminate randomness in your life.
- List ways to stay more present.

_____

_____

_____

_____

_____

_____

_____

_____

_____

_____

Feelings without honesty are defenses.
The world without honesty is an illusion.
Memory without honesty is only a fantasy.
Time without honesty can never be now.
Space without honesty can never be here.
Love without honesty is possessiveness.

Without honesty there is no real growth.
Without honesty there is no real freedom.
Without honesty there is no hope.
Without honesty nothing is real.
Without honesty nothing is.

— **Author Unknown**

Resource Guide

Clutter/Organizing/Self-Care

Aslett, Don, *Clutter's Last Stand*, F&W Pub., 1984;
Clutter Free, March Creek Press, 1995

Bridges, Carol, *The Medicine Woman's Guide to Being in Business for Yourself*, Earth Nation Publishing, 1992

Burka, Jane & Yuen, Lenora, *Procrastination: Why You Do It, What To Do About It*, Addison Wesley, 1983

Campbell, Jeff, *Clutter Control*, Dell, 1992

Covey, Steven R, *The Seven Habits of Highly Effective People*, Fireside, 1989

Cox, Connie & Evatt,Cris, *Simply Organized*, Berkley, 1998

Eisenberg, Ronni & Kelly, Kate, *Organize Your Home*, Hyperion, 1994

Felton, Sandra, *The New Messies Manual*, Revell, 1999.

Kingston, Karen, *Clear Your Clutter With Feng Shui*, Broadway, 1999

Knaus,William J., Ed.D., *Do It Now! Break The Procrastination Habit*, Wiley, 1998

Morgenstern, Julie, *Organizing from the Inside Out*, Holt, 1998

Orman, Suze, *The Courage to Be Rich*, Riverhead Books, 1999

Passoff, Michelle, *Lighten Up*, Harper Perennial, 1998

St. James, Elaine, *Living the Simple Life*, Hyperion, 1996

Winston, Stephanie, *Getting Organized*, Warner, 1991;
Getting Out From Under, Perseus, 1999

Living Simply
Shi, David, *The Simple Life*, Oxford, 1985
St. James, Elaine, *Living the Simple Life*, Hyperion, 1996

Feng Shui
Bridges, Carol, *A Soul in Place, Reclaiming Home as Sacred Space*, Earth Nation Pub., 1995
Collins, Terah Kathryn, *The Western Guide to Feng Shui*, Hay House, Inc., 1996
Kennedy, David Daniel, *Feng Shui Tips for a Better Life*, Storey Books, 1998

Catalogs
Organized 800-803-9400
Hard to Find Tools 800-926-7000
The Container Store 800-733-3532
Alston's 800-447-0048
Lillian Vernon 800-545-5426
William's Sonoma 800-541-2233
Hold Everything 800-421-2264

> These are all wonderful catalogs, yet they will begin to inundate you every few months. If you don't want this to happen, get one and tell them to take you off their mailing list immediately. It will take a few issues, and then they will stop.

Journals
Simple Living 206-464-4800
Qi-Journal of Health & Fitness
    Box 18476, Anaheim, CA 92817

Internet under **Feng Shui** — Patricia J. Santhuff

Magazines
*Family Circle, Woman's Day, Country Living
Natural Home* 800-340-5846

Creating The Healthy Home
The Bau-Biologie Institute 813-461-4371

Helpful Addresses and Ideas
National Association of Professional Organizers
1033 La Posada Dr., Austin, TX 78752
512-206-0151

Mail Preference Service
POB 9008, Farmingdale, NY 22735-9008
They will take your name off junk mail lists.

Send for this booklet for $3.00, *Stop Junk Mail Forever* by
Marc Eisensen from Good Advice Press,
Elizaville, NY, 12523 — 914-458-1400

Sandra Felton's Self-Help Group
Messies Anonymous, 5025 S.W. 114 Avenue
Miami, FL 33165
She also has a booklet on *The Packrat Syndrome*. To
order call 800-MESS AWAY.

The OCD Foundation
POB 9573, New Haven, CT 06535
OCD WebServer: www. fairlite.com/ocd/

The Anxiety Disorders Assoc. of America
6000 Executive Blvd., Suite 200
Rockville, M 20852-3081 — 301-231-9350.

Important: Be aware that when you send for
catalogs, receive magazine and journal
subscriptions, join professional organizations, deal
with auto insurance and credit bureaus, they will
and can sell your name to other mailing lists. Ask or
write them the following: **"Do not lease, sell, or
trade my name or address."**

The Post Office also sells your name to junk mail
distributors when you submit any change of address
to them.

Some of the fine authors who have written on self-esteem are:

Wayne Dyer
John Bradshaw
Louise Hay
John Gray
Arnold M. Patent
Charles L. Whitfield, M.D.
Julia Cameron

We are caught in an escapable network
of mutuality, tied in a single garment
of destiny. Whatever affects one
directly affects all indirectly.

—Martin Luther King